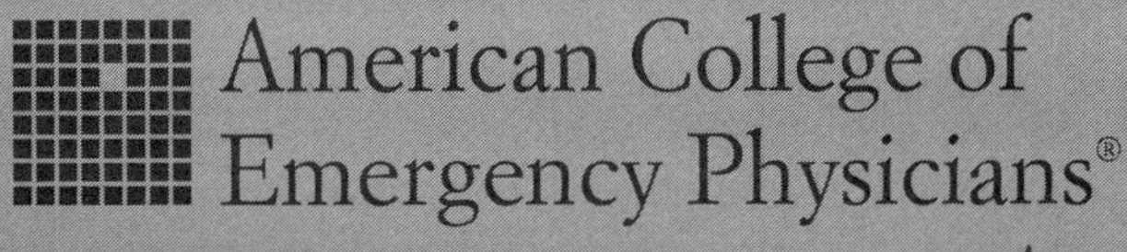

eACLS™ Study Guide,

SECOND EDITION

Stephen J. Rahm, NREMT-P

JONES AND BARTLETT PUBLISHERS
Sudbury, Massachusetts
BOSTON TORONTO LONDON SINGAPORE

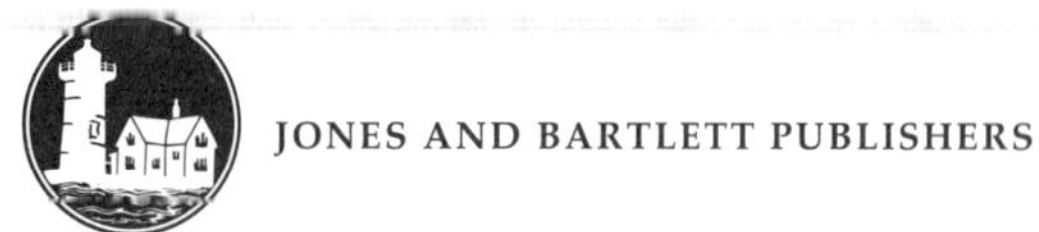

World Headquarters
40 Tall Pine Drive
Sudbury, MA 01776
978-443-5000
info@jbpub.com
www.jbpub.com

Jones and Bartlett Publishers Canada
6339 Ormindale Way
Mississauga, ON L5V 1J2
CANADA

Jones and Bartlett Publishers International
Barb House, Barb Mews
London W6 7PA
UK

Production Credits
Chief Executive Officer: Clayton Jones
Chief Operating Officer: Donald W. Jones, Jr.
President, Higher Education and Professional Publishing: Robert W. Holland, Jr.
V.P., Sales and Marketing: William J. Kane
V.P., Production and Design: Anne Spencer
V.P., Manufacturing and Inventory Control: Therese Connell
Publisher, Public Safety Group: Kimberly Brophy
Publisher: Lawrence D. Newell
Production Editor: Jenny Corriveau
Cover and Text Design: Kristin Ohlin
Cover Image: © Brad Wrobleski/Masterfile
Compositor: Auburn Associates, Inc.
Printing and Binding: Courier Stoughton

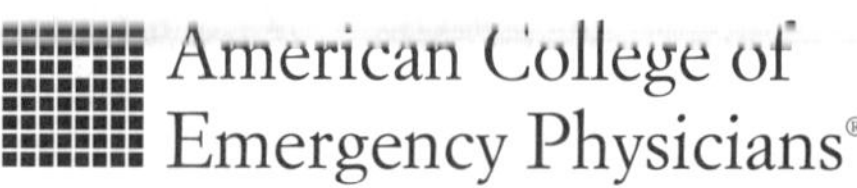

ADVANCING EMERGENCY CARE

1125 Executive Circle
Post Office Box 619911
Dallas, TX 75261-9911
800-798-1822
www.acep.org

Marta Foster, Director, Educational and Professional Publications

Tom Werlinich, Associate Executive Director, Educational and Professional Products Division

ISBN-13: 978-0-7637-4954-5

ISBN-10: 0-7637-4954-0

6048

Jones and Bartlett's books and products are available through most bookstores and online booksellers. To contact Jones and Bartlett Publishers directly, call 800-832-0034, fax 978-443-8000, or visit our website www.jbpub.com.

Substantial discounts on bulk quantities of Jones and Bartlett's publications are available to corporations, professional associations, and other qualified organizations. For details and specific discount information, contact the special sales department at Jones and Bartlett via the above contact information or send an email to specialsales@jbpub.com.

Figures 1-3–1-21, 3-1–3-5, 3-10–3-13, 4-1–4-12, and illustrations on pages 79-80, 83, 106, 107, 111, 114, 115, are from *Arrhythmia Recognition: The Art of Interpretation* and *12-Lead ECG: The Art of Interpretation,* Courtesy of Tomas B. Garcia, MD.

Reviewed by the American College of Emergency Physicians

The American College of Emergency Physicians (ACEP) makes every effort to ensure that its product and program reviewers are knowledgeable content experts and recognized authorities in their fields. Readers are nevertheless advised that the statements and opinions expressed in this publication are provided as guidelines and should not be construed as College policy unless specifically referred to as such. The College disclaims any liability or responsibility for the consequences of any actions taken in reliance on those statements or opinions. The materials contained herein are not intended to establish policy, procedure, or a standard of care. To contact ACEP write to: PO Box 619911, Dallas, TX 75261-9911; call toll-free 800-798-1822, touch 6, or 972-550-0911.

This textbook is intended solely as a guide to the appropriate procedures to be employed when rendering emergency care to the sick and injured. It is not intended as a statement of the standards of care required in any particular situation, because circumstances and the patient's physical condition can vary widely from one emergency to another. Nor is it intended that this textbook shall in any way advise emergency personnel concerning legal authority to perform the activities or procedures discussed. Such local determinations should be made only with the aid of legal counsel.

Printed in the United States of America
11 10 09 08 07 10 9 8 7 6 5 4 3 2

CONTENTS

Introduction

Welcome to eACLS™! The "e" refers to **e**lectronic and **e**asy. ACLS refers to Advanced Cardiac Life Support. This study guide has been developed to assist you, the ACLS provider or instructor, in reviewing the principles and concepts of managing a patient with a respiratory or cardiovascular system emergency. The information and activities in this study guide are intended to accommodate both those who are relatively new to ACLS and the experienced provider.

The eACLS™ Study Guide is the required student manual for those completing the eACLS™ initial or refresher classroom-based course. It is not required for those completing the eACLS™ online course, but does provide additional support for online course students. The eACLS™ course and this study guide provide you with the opportunity to review your baseline knowledge of the following key components of advanced cardiac care:

- Cardiac rhythms
- Pharmacologic therapy
- Electrical therapy
- Patient assessment

Specific practice cases are presented in this study guide and the eACLS™ course that incorporate the above key components. These cases include:

- Acute coronary syndromes (ACS)
- Asystole
- Automated external defibrillation
- Bradycardia
- Pulseless electrical activity
- Respiratory arrest
- Stroke
- Tachycardia—narrow complex
- Tachycardia—wide complex
- Ventricular fibrillation

Each case will present a patient, the patient's chief complaint, the ECG tracing if applicable, and the initial examination findings. After being provided with this information, you must decide which treatment algorithm/approach would be most appropriate for the patient.

Within each case, you will be asked questions about the assessment and treatment that you would provide for the patient. More challenging questions will be identified as **"Beyond eACLS Basics."** A summary, which contains the answers and rationales for the practice case questions, will immediately follow each practice case.

At the end of this study guide, you will find a comprehensive practice written examination, which has 50 randomly developed items from all 10 of the eACLS™ cases. The answers, along with rationales for both correct and incorrect responses, will immediately follow the practice written examination.

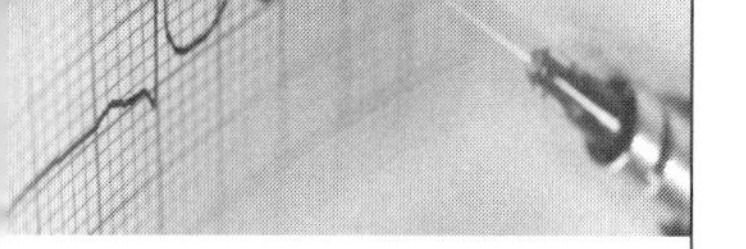

More about eACLS

eACLS™ is a highly interactive program that allows healthcare professionals to show their competency, as well as earn national certification, as an ACLS provider.

Each of the eACLS™ case studies has the following components:

- Case introduction known as "Your Patient," which covers your initial patient presentation
- Assessment tutorial
- Treatment tutorial
- Interactivities with multiple-choice, fill-in-the-blank, and matching exercises that assess your understanding of the key concepts for each case
- Case summary
- A highly interactive, video-based case simulation, which puts you in the driver's seat of assessing and managing the patient

You must successfully complete all of these components in each case before you will be able to move on to another case.

After completing the necessary didactic and practical skills for eACLS™, you must pass a comprehensive 50-item, multiple-choice written examination. If you fail to achieve the minimum score of 84% on the first examination, additional opportunities are provided using alternative examinations that evaluate the same content and have the same degree of difficulty.

Feel free to use this study guide as a preparatory tool for eACLS™ as well as a reference tool during the program itself. We are confident that you will find eACLS™ to be an interactive experience that is both fun and educational.

Chapter 1

Review of Cardiac Rhythms

Introduction

This chapter focuses primarily on the cardiac rhythms addressed in eACLS and is not intended to be inclusive of all cardiac rhythms that could be encountered by the health care provider. Clinicians are encouraged to refer to the text *Arrhythmia Recognition: The Art of Interpretation* by Tomas B. Garcia, MD, and Geoffrey T. Miller, NREMT-P (Jones and Bartlett Publishers, 2004) for a detailed review of the cardiac electrical conduction system, including all cardiac rhythm disturbances and their variants.

Although it is important to identify the specific cardiac rhythm disturbance presenting on the electrocardiogram (ECG), it is equally, if not more, important to recognize whether or not the patient is stable or unstable as a result of the cardiac rhythm disturbance. This status determines the most appropriate treatment approach.

This chapter reviews the following:

Cardiac Electrical Conduction System
- Conduction system components
- ECG waveform representations
- Normal sinus rhythm (NSR)

ECG Markers of Acute Coronary Syndrome
- ST-segment depression and elevation
- T-wave inversion
- Q waves

Bradycardias
- Sinus bradycardia
- Idioventricular rhythm
- Heart blocks

Tachycardias
- Narrow QRS complex
  - Sinus tachycardia
  - Supraventricular tachycardia (SVT)
  - Atrial fibrillation
  - Atrial flutter
- Wide QRS complex
  - Monomorphic ventricular tachycardia
  - Polymorphic ventricular tachycardia

Cardiac Arrest Rhythms
- Ventricular fibrillation/pulseless ventricular tachycardia
- Asystole
- Pulseless electrical activity (PEA)

Cardiac Electrical Conduction System

Conduction System Components

As you will recall, the myocardium is a muscle unlike no other in the human body. It has the ability to generate its own electricity, a process called *automaticity.* Through a specialized conduction system, electrical impulses are generated by a pacemaker and then transmitted, in an organized fashion, throughout the myocardium (Figure 1-1). A pacemaker is a collection of nerve fibers that sets the inherent rate of electrical discharge for the heart.

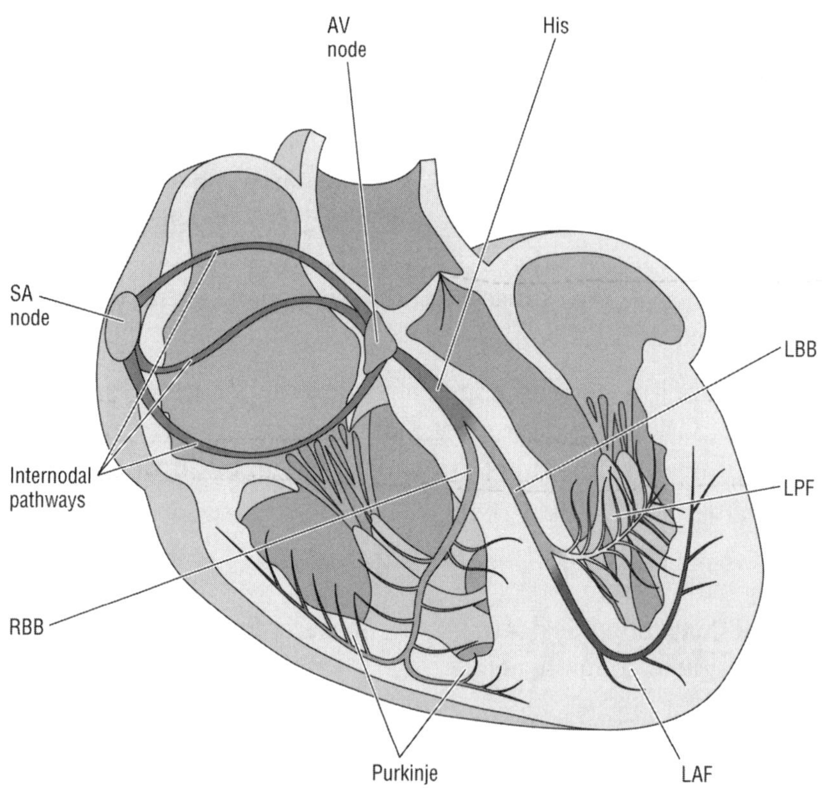

Figure 1-1: Cardiac conduction system.

In the normal heart, the primary pacemaker is the sinoatrial (SA) node, also referred to as the sinus node. The SA node is located in the superior aspect of the right atrium and inherently discharges 60–100 electrical impulses per minute.

Once initiated in the SA node, the electrical impulse travels, via the internodal pathways, throughout the right and left atria and depolarizes their cells. This depolarization (electrical discharge) stimulates the atrial muscle to contract.

The impulse travels farther to the atrioventricular (AV) node, where it is briefly delayed before entering the ventricles. This delay is necessary to allow the atria and

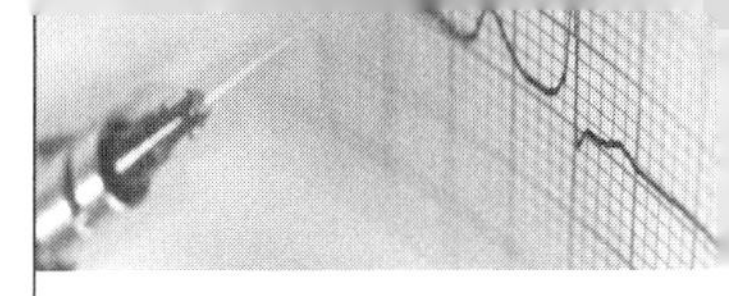

ventricles to beat independently of each other, thus functioning as a double pump. The AV node is located in the wall of the right atrium.

If for some reason the SA node fails as the primary pacemaker, the AV node can assume the responsibility. However, it does so at a slower pace, with an inherent discharge rate of 40–60 electrical impulses per minute. After the brief AV nodal delay, the impulse travels through the bundle of His, which is the only route of electrical transmission between the atria and the ventricles.

The bundle of His, which is located partially in the walls of the right atrium and in the interventricular septum, gives rise to a right and left bundle branch, the left of which has an anterior and a posterior fascicle. It only makes sense that the left bundle branch has two fascicles because the left ventricle is much larger than the right ventricle. The bundle branches terminate into the Purkinje system, which depolarizes the ventricular cells, thus causing the ventricular muscle to contract.

If both the SA and the AV nodes fail to generate an electrical impulse, the ventricles can become the primary pacemaker; however, they generate electricity much slower, at a rate of only 20–40 electrical impulses per minute.

ECG Waveform Representations

Each event in the cardiac conduction system produces a specific waveform that can be analyzed with an ECG. One entire cardiac cycle produces a single complex of waveforms (Figure 1-2). It is important to remember that the ECG is *not* a representation of myocardial mechanics; it merely depicts the electrical events that stimulate myocardial contraction. A rhythm on the ECG is not equivalent to a palpable pulse.

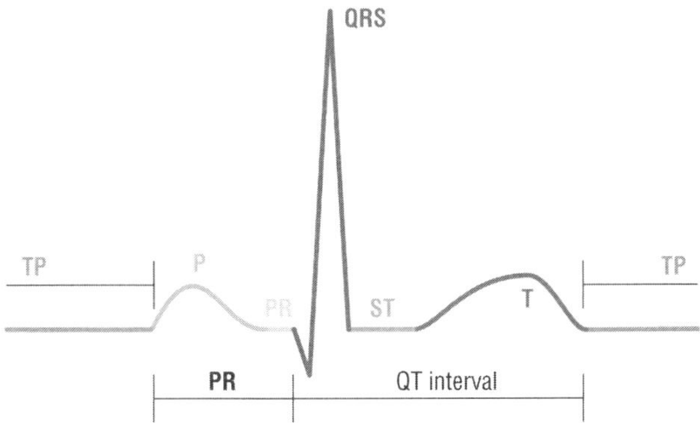

Figure 1-2: ECG complex waveforms.

The P wave, which is normally upright, is the first waveform on the ECG. It represents simultaneous depolarization of both atria. The P-R segment, which is the time frame between the end of the P wave and the beginning of the QRS complex, represents the delay at the AV node. The P-R interval, which begins at the initiation of the P wave and ends at the QRS complex, represents the entire atrial depolarization process, including the delay at the AV node.

Collectively, the QRS complex represents ventricular depolarization. The Q wave, which is the first negative deflection after the P wave, can be present or absent. Q-wave significance is discussed in the next section of this chapter. The R wave is the first positive deflection after the P wave. The S wave is the first negative deflection after the R wave.

The ST segment represents the time frame between ventricular depolarization and repolarization. The ST segment should be isoelectric, which is the baseline of the cardiac cycle in which there is electrical neutrality. ST-segment depression or elevation of less than 1 mm may be insignificant; however, this is not conclusive. ST-segment depression and elevation are discussed in the next section of this chapter.

The T wave, which represents ventricular repolarization, is the first deflection that occurs after the ST segment. The T-wave deflection should be in the same direction as the QRS complex. T-wave inversion is also discussed in the next section of this chapter.

Normal Sinus Rhythm (NSR)

Now that we have reviewed the cardiac electrical conduction system and the ECG waveforms that it represents, let's look at a normal sinus rhythm. In order to recognize the abnormal, we must first recognize and appreciate the normal. A normal sinus rhythm (Figure 1-3) would indicate that all components of the cardiac conduction system are intact and are functioning normally. Remember, it does not mean that the patient is stable or even has a pulse.

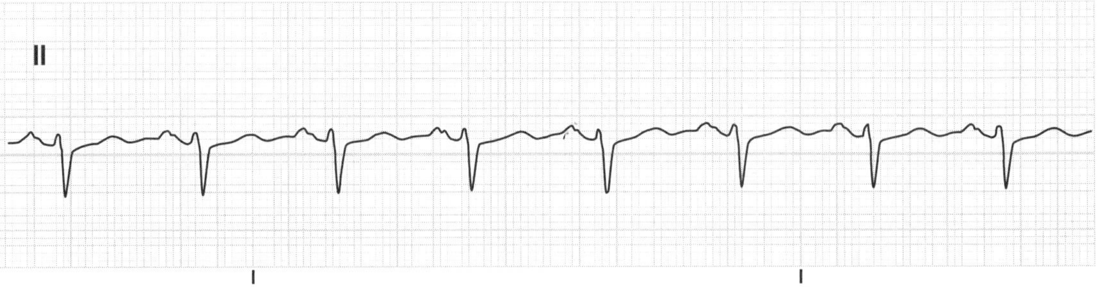

Figure 1-3: Normal sinus rhythm.

Rhythm: Regular

Rate: 60–100 beats/minute

P waves: Present and upright

P-R Interval: 0.12–0.20 seconds, consistent

QRS Complex: 0.06–0.12 seconds

P wave to QRS ratio: 1 to 1

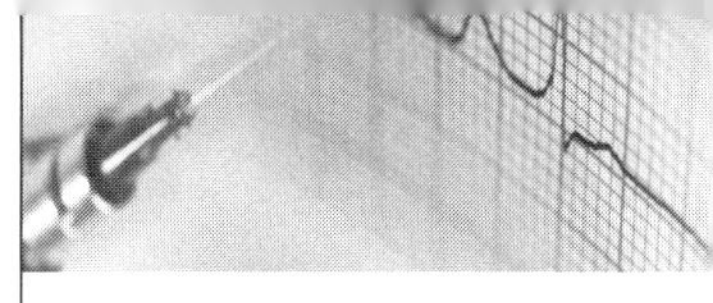

Origin

Normal sinus rhythm indicates that the SA node is the primary pacemaker site and that all components of the cardiac electrical conduction system are intact and functioning normally.

Clinical Significance

None, unless it occurs in the absence of a pulse.

ECG Markers of Acute Coronary Syndrome

ST-Segment Depression and Elevation

The ST segment represents the time frame between ventricular depolarization and repolarization. It should be at the isoelectric line, or the period of time when the myocardium is electrically neutral.

Although slight depression and elevation of the ST segment in various lead configurations may be benign, we must assume that any ST-segment depression or elevation in a patient with chest pain or other signs and symptoms of an acute coronary syndrome is significant and is representative of acute myocardial ischemia or infarction until proved otherwise (Figure 1-4).

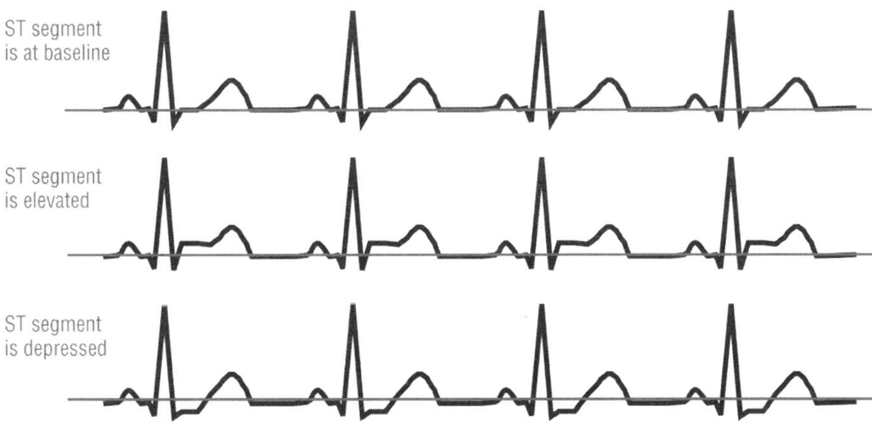

Figure 1-4: ST segment changes.

As a general rule, ST-segment depression is indicative of myocardial ischemia, and ST-segment elevation indicates myocardial injury. For these findings to be conclusive, one would need a 12-lead ECG tracing because these changes would be clinically significant if they were observed in at least two contiguous leads. This is not an observation that we can make with a standard cardiac monitor, which views only one lead.

When the patient with an acute coronary syndrome is managed, a 12-lead ECG is clearly indicated in order to aid in the diagnosis of myocardial ischemia or infarction so that the most appropriate reperfusion strategy (e.g., thrombolytics, angioplasty) can be selected. Although 12-lead electrocardiography is beyond the scope of this study guide, we must remember that patients with a normal 12-lead ECG can be having an acute coronary syndrome. This reminds us of that ever so important concept of "treating the patient, not the monitor."

T-Wave Inversion

The T wave represents repolarization of the ventricles. Its deflection should be in the same direction as the QRS complex. An inverted T wave (Figure 1-5) can indicate myocardial ischemia. Again, for this finding to be conclusive, a 12-lead ECG would be required for the T waves to be viewed in other leads.

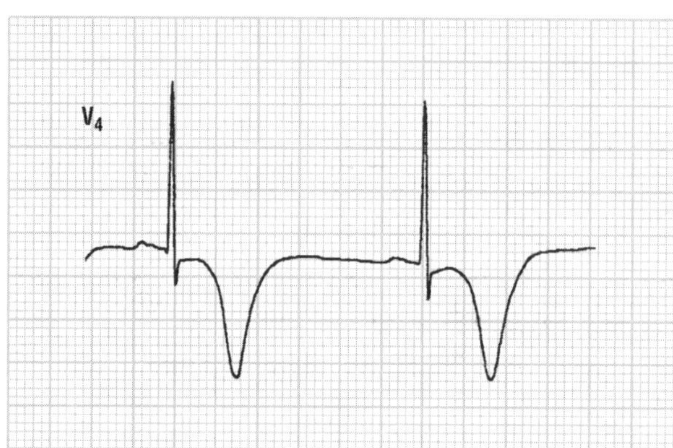

Figure 1-5: T-wave inversion.

As with changes in the ST segment, we must assume that T-wave inversion in a patient with signs and symptoms of an acute coronary syndrome is clinically significant until proven otherwise.

Q Waves

The Q wave, if visible, is the first negative deflection after the P wave. Q waves can be insignificant in some leads. However, this is not a safe assumption to make if they are seen on an ECG in a patient with chest pain.

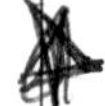

A significant or "pathologic" Q wave is defined as one that is either one third the total height of the QRS complex (Figure 1-6), or more than 0.03 seconds wide (Figure 1-7).

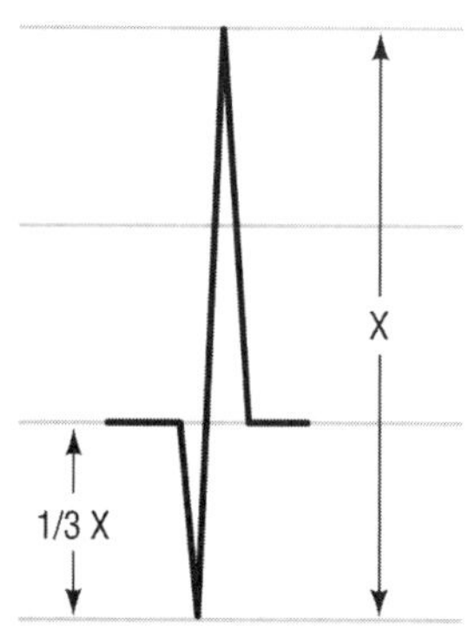

Figure 1-6: Q-wave height.

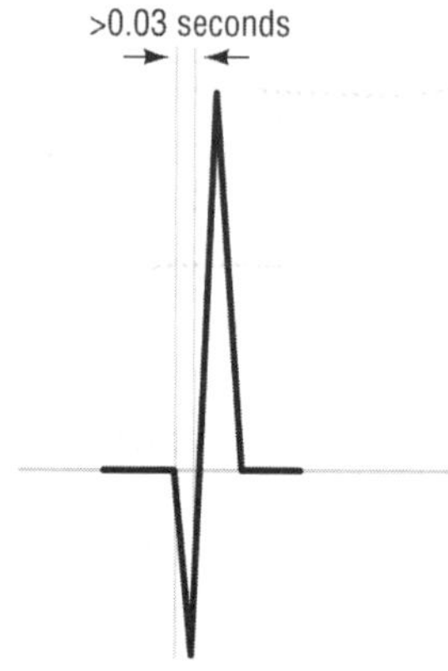

Figure 1-7: Q-wave width.

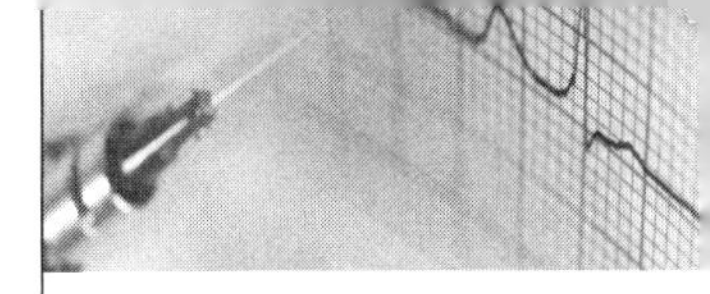

Pathologic Q waves represent dead myocardium and are the ECG signature of a myocardial infarction. Without the benefit of a previous 12-lead ECG tracing, one cannot conclude the age of the infarct. In the best interest of the patient, any Q wave should be considered to be an acute myocardial infarction in progress, especially if it is accompanied by ST-segment elevation.

Bradycardias

Introduction

Bradycardia, as defined by a heart rate of less than 60 beats per minute, can result in a decrease in cardiac output, which would make the patient clinically unstable. Absolute bradycardia refers to any heart rate that is less than 60 beats per minute (Figure 1-8). Relative bradycardia occurs when the heart rate is faster than expected (may be greater than 60 beats per minute) and is accompanied by serious signs and symptoms (e.g., hypotension, altered mental status).

Sinus Bradycardia

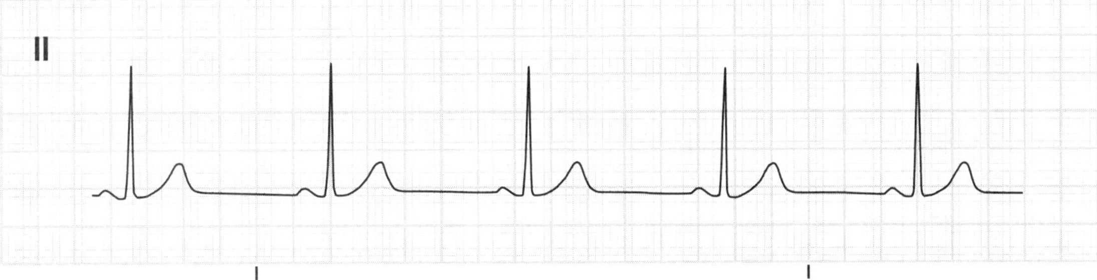

Figure 1-8: Sinus bradycardia.

Rhythm: Regular

Rate: Less than 60 beats/minute

P waves: Present and normal

P-R Interval: 0.12–0.20 seconds, consistent

QRS Complex: 0.06–0.12 seconds

P wave to QRS ratio: 1 to 1

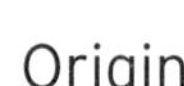

Origin

Sinus bradycardia results from excess vagal stimulation, which slows sinoatrial (SA) node discharge. Other causes include disease or damage to the cardiac electrical conduction system as well as the effect of certain drugs (e.g., beta blockers).

Clinical Significance

Sinus bradycardia can result in a decreased cardiac output. In well-conditioned athletes, sinus bradycardia may be a normal finding.

Idioventricular Rhythm

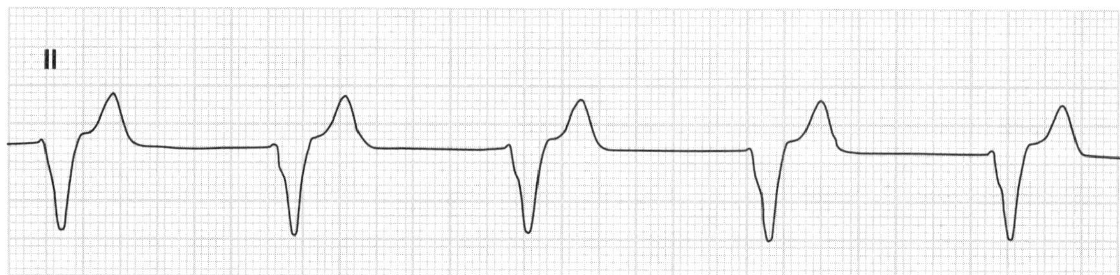

Figure 1-9: Idioventricular rhythm.

Rhythm: Regular

Rate: 20–40 beats/minute

P waves: None

P-R Interval: None

QRS Complex: Greater than 0.12 seconds, bizarre appearance

P wave to QRS ratio: None

Origin

Idioventricular rhythms (Figure 1-9) occur when a ventricular focus acts as the primary pacemaker for the heart. This is evidenced by the wide and bizarre appearance of the QRS complexes and the slow ventricular rate. Because atrial activity is absent, there are no P waves.

Clinical Significance

In the absence of atrial contraction, minimal volumes of blood are ejected into the ventricles. Additionally, because the ventricular rate is so slow, the cardiac output is significantly decreased.

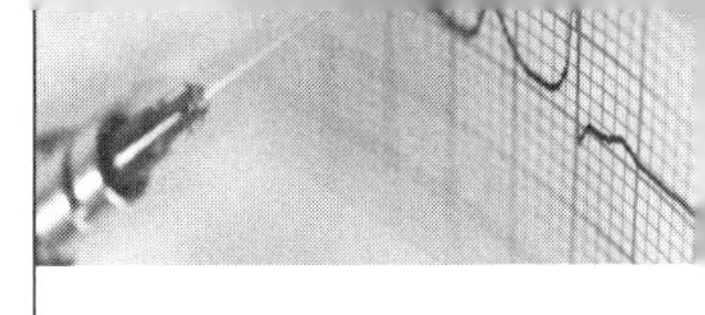

Heart Blocks

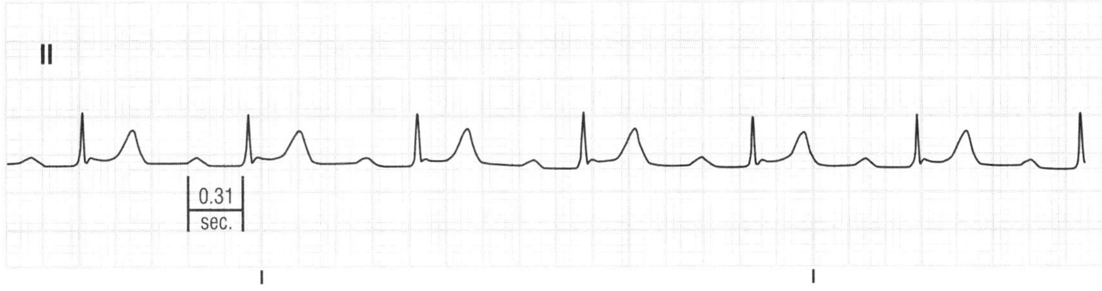

Figure 1-10: First-degree AV block.

Rhythm: Regular

Rate: Normal or slow

P waves: Present and normal

P-R Interval: Prolonged greater than 0.20 seconds

QRS Complex: 0.06–0.12 seconds

P wave to QRS ratio: 1 to 1

Origin

First-degree AV block (Figure 1-10) is caused by an abnormal delay at the AV node, which prolongs the P-R interval longer than 0.20 seconds. Factors such as vagal stimulation, AV nodal disease, and certain medications can cause this cardiac rhythm.

Clinical Significance

Unlike the higher-degree AV blocks, first-degree AV block is less frequently associated with bradycardia. However, when first-degree AV block is associated with bradycardia, cardiac output can fall. First-degree AV block may be a normal variant in some people.

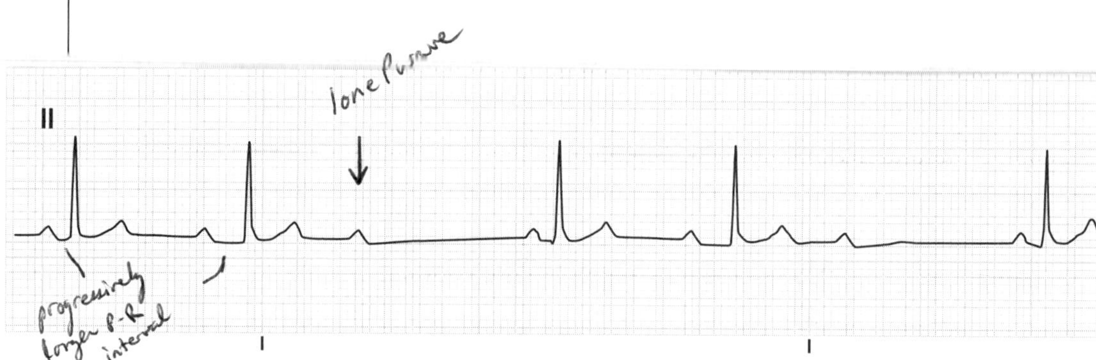

Figure 1-11: Second-degree AV block Type I.

Rhythm: Regularly irregular

Rate: Normal or slow

P waves: Present and normal

P-R Interval: Progressively lengthened until a QRS complex is dropped

QRS Complex: 0.06–0.12 seconds

P wave to QRS ratio: Variable: 2:1, 3:1, 4:1, etc.

Origin

Second-degree AV block type I (Figure 1-11) is caused by AV nodal disease or vagal stimulation. Each complex is progressively delayed at the AV node until a complex is completely blocked, which results in a "stand alone" P wave without a QRS complex.

Clinical Significance

Depending on the degree of block (e.g. 2:1, 3:1, 4:1), this cardiac rhythm can either present with a normal or a bradycardic rate. If second-degree AV block is associated with bradycardia, cardiac output may decrease.

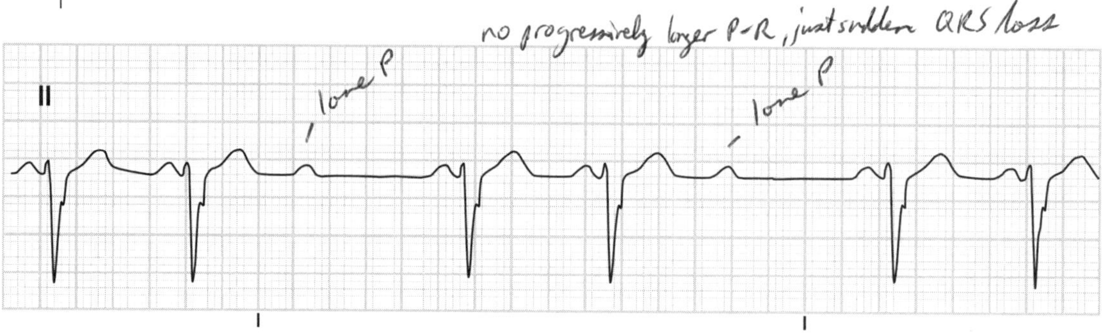

Figure 1-12: Second-degree AV block type II.

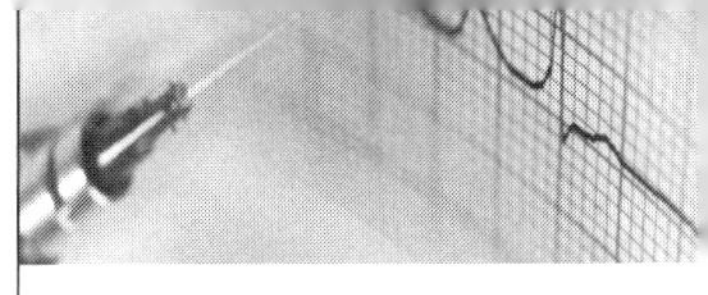

Rhythm: Variable, depending on the P:QRS ratio

Rate: Variable, but generally slow

P waves: Present and normal

P-R Interval: 0.12–0.20 seconds of the normally conducted complexes

QRS Complex: 0.06–0.12 seconds

P wave to QRS ratio: Variable: 2:1, 3:1, 4:1, etc.

Origin

Second-degree AV block type II (Figure 1-12) occurs when the AV node intermittently blocks some of the atrial conducted complexes. This results in some P waves that are not followed by a QRS complex.

Clinical Significance

Second-degree AV block type II results from more severe AV nodal disease or excessive vagal tone. It is frequently associated with bradycardia, which can decrease cardiac output.

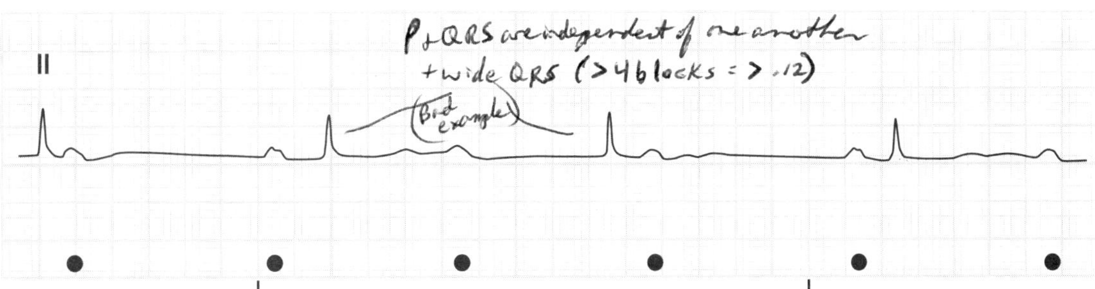

Figure 1-13: Third-degree AV block.

Rhythm: Regular

Rate: 20–40 beats/minute

P-waves: Present and normal

P-R Interval: Variable, no pattern

QRS Complex: Usually greater than 0.12 seconds

P-wave to QRS ratio: Variable

Origin

Third-degree AV block (Figure 1-13) occurs as the result of a complete block at the AV node. Complete blockage at the AV node does not allow any of the atrial conducted complexes to enter the ventricles. As a result, the ventricles respond with escape complexes, thus producing a wide QRS complex. Third-degree AV block is also referred to as *complete heart block.*

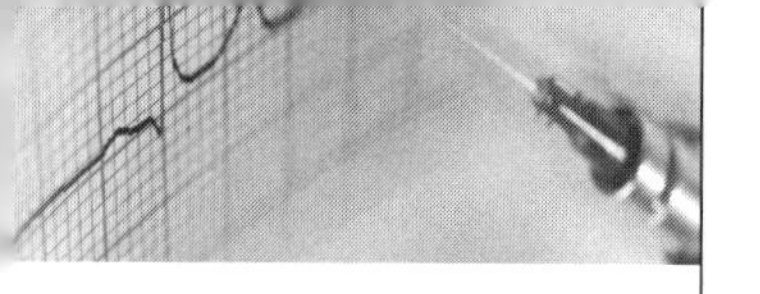

Clinical Significance

Because atrial and ventricular contractions are dissociated, cardiac output is significantly decreased and the patient is almost always clinically unstable. Because the atrial conducted complexes cannot traverse the AV node and enter the ventricles, a ventricular pacemaker initiates an impulse at its inherent rate of 20–40 beats per minute, which produces wide QRS complexes and makes the rhythm severely bradycardic.

Tachycardias

Introduction

Tachycardia is defined as a heart rate that is greater than 100 beats per minute. This section discusses both narrow and wide complex tachycardias. If the heart beats too fast, the ventricles may not adequately fill. This would result in a decrease in cardiac output, making the patient clinically unstable. In this section, we review tachycardias that have narrow or wide QRS complexes.

Narrow QRS Complex

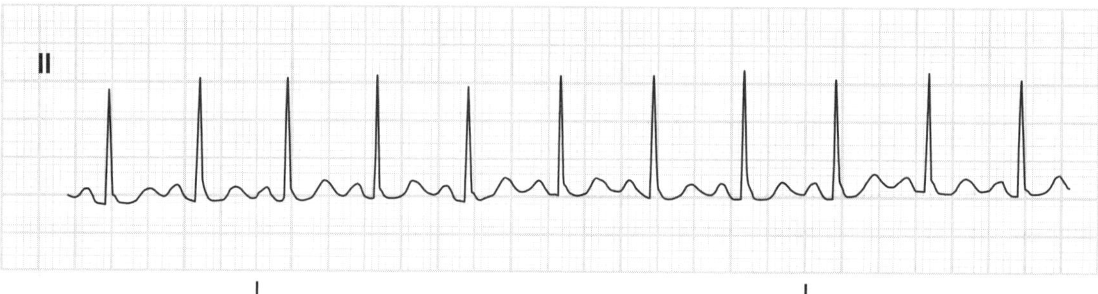

Figure 1-14: Sinus tachycardia.

Rhythm: Regular

Rate: 100–150 beats/minute

P waves: Present and normal

P-R Interval: 0.12–0.20 seconds

QRS Complex: 0.06–0.12 seconds

P wave to QRS ratio: 1 to 1

Origin

Sinus tachycardia (Figure 1-14) occurs when the SA node discharges faster than its inherent rate of 60–100 electrical impulses per minute. This can be caused by certain medications or by situations that require an increase in cardiac output (e.g., shock, fever, hypoxemia, exercise).

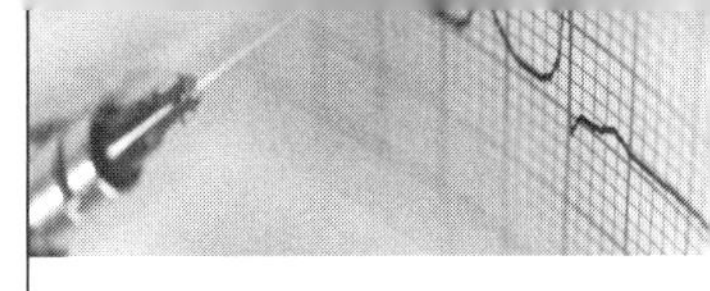

Clinical Significance

Sinus tachycardia can result in a decreased cardiac output secondary to inadequate ventricular filling.

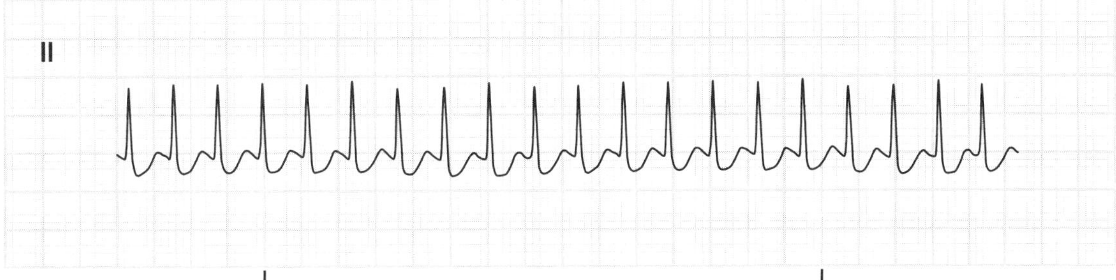

Figure 1-15: Supraventricular tachycardia (SVT).

The term *supraventricular* tachycardia (SVT) (Figure 1-15) can encompass a variety of cardiac rhythms, including atrial tachycardia, ectopic atrial tachycardia, rapid atrial fibrillation or flutter, and junctional tachycardia. For the purposes of this review, we define SVT as being any narrow-complex tachycardia with a heart rate that exceeds 150 beats per minute.

Rhythm: Regular

Rate: Greater than 150 beats/minute

P waves: Present but may not be visible because of the rapid ventricular rate

P-R Interval: Usually not measurable

QRS Complex: 0.06–0.12 seconds

P wave to QRS ratio: Usually unable to determine because of the rapid ventricular rate

Origin

Supraventricular tachycardia occurs when a supraventricular (above the ventricles) pacemaker initiates the cardiac cycle. This pacemaker is not necessarily the SA node. Like sinus tachycardia, SVT can be caused by certain medications or situations that require an increase in cardiac output (e.g., shock, fever, hypoxemia, exercise) as well as disease of the SA node.

Clinical Significance

Supraventricular tachycardia can result in a decreased cardiac output secondary to inadequate ventricular filling, more so than sinus tachycardia.

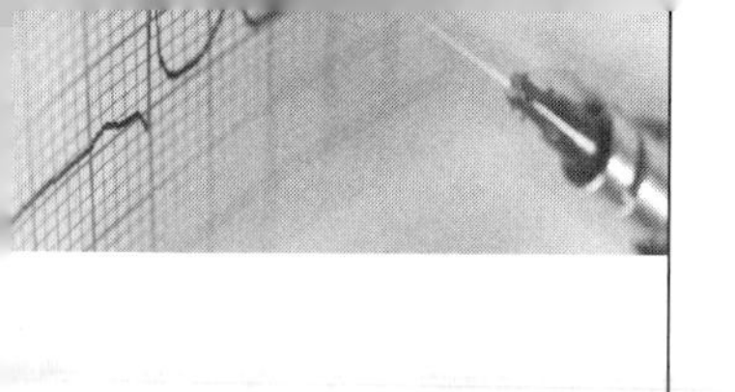

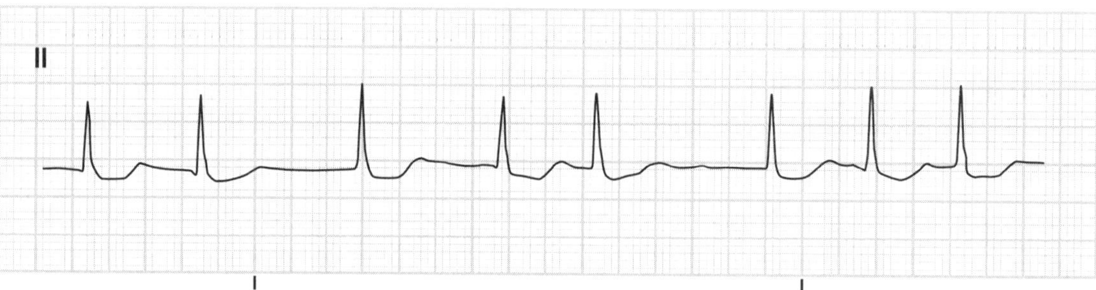

Figure 1-16: Atrial fibrillation.

Rhythm: Irregularly irregular

Rate: Variable, ventricular rate can be fast or slow

P waves: None, only fibrillatory waves

P-R Interval: None

QRS Complex: 0.06–0.12 seconds

P wave to QRS ratio: None

Origin

Atrial fibrillation (Figure 1-16) is the result of multiple atrial pacemakers discharging chaotically. As a result, there are no discernable P waves, but rather fibrillatory waves between each QRS complex. Because there is no coordinated electrical pattern from the atria to the ventricles, electricity traverses the AV node sporadically, resulting in a ventricular rhythm that is irregularly irregular.

Clinical Significance

Atrial fibrillation is frequently encountered in patients with congestive heart failure or in those with damage or disease of the SA node. Several potential problems are associated with this arrhythmia. First, because the atria are fibrillating, blood has a tendency to stagnate, which increases the risk of microemboli formation and subsequent pulmonary, coronary, or cerebral embolism. Second, when the ventricular rate of atrial fibrillation exceeds 100 beats per minute, cardiac output can decrease. This decrease in cardiac output is compounded by decreased atrial kick because smaller volumes of blood are ejected into the ventricles from the fibrillating atria.

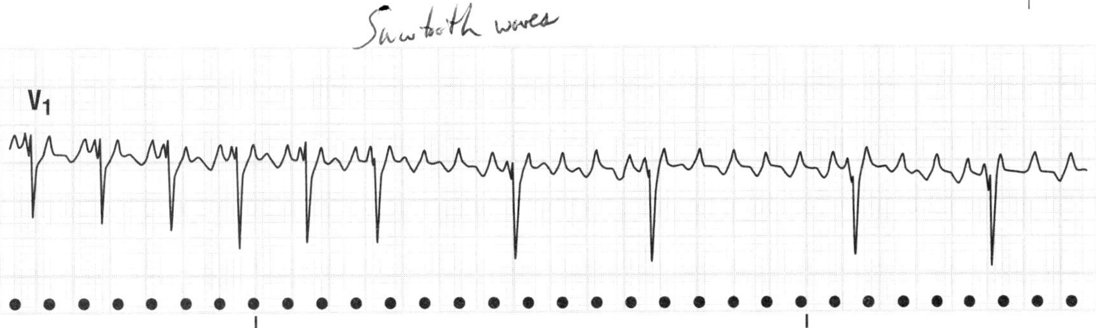

Figure 1-17: Atrial flutter.

Rhythm: Variable, depending on the ratio of F waves to QRS complexes

Rate: Variable

P waves: Saw-toothed appearance, flutter (F) waves

P-R Interval: Variable

QRS Complex: 0.06–0.12 seconds

P wave to QRS ratio: Variable, but most commonly 2 to 1

Origin

Atrial flutter (Figure 1-17) is the result of an ectopic atrial pacemaker outside of the SA node. The ectopic pacemaker is commonly in the lower atrium, near the AV node. SA node function is completely suppressed by atrial flutter. Instead of P waves, atrial flutter produces flutter (F) waves, which represent abnormal atrial depolarization that commonly begins near the AV node and progresses across the atria in a retrograde direction.

Clinical Significance

Atrial flutter also occurs in patients with congestive heart failure and in those with damage or disease of the SA node. As with atrial fibrillation, complications occur with this arrhythmia as a result of inadequate ventricular filling, especially when it is accompanied by a rapid ventricular rate. Cardiac output can significantly decrease.

Wide QRS Complex

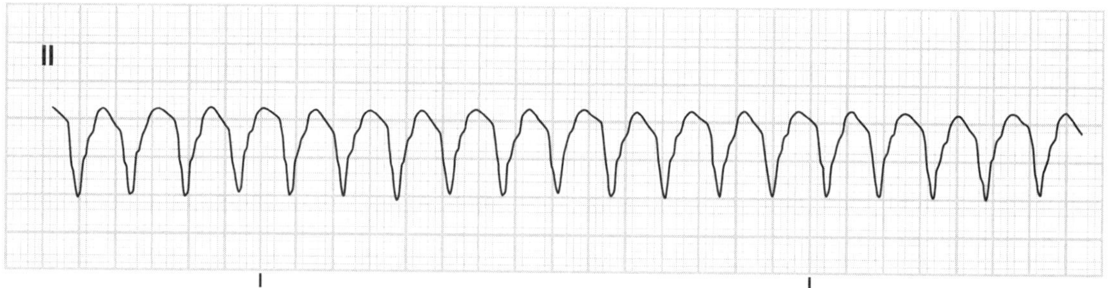

Figure 1-18: Monomorphic ventricular tachycardia.

Rhythm: Regular, may be slightly irregular

Rate: 100–200 beats/minute

P waves: None, occasional P waves may be seen in the QRS complexes

P-R Interval: None

QRS Complex: Greater than 0.12 seconds, wide and bizarre

P wave to QRS ratio: None

Origin

Monomorphic ventricular tachycardia (Figure 1-18), which is the most common form of this rhythm, has complexes that are all of the same shape, size, and direction. It is caused by an ectopic pacemaker site in the ventricle, which, in effect, overrides atrial activity. Although occasional P waves may be seen, they occur infrequently and are buried in the wide, bizarre QRS complexes.

Clinical Significance

Ventricular tachycardia can be the result of many underlying causes, the most common of which are significant coronary artery disease, QT interval prolongation, and electrolyte imbalance, specifically potassium. In ventricular tachycardia, the atria do not contract regularly, therefore, the ventricles do not adequately fill with blood before they contract. This results in a marked reduction in stroke volume and cardiac output.

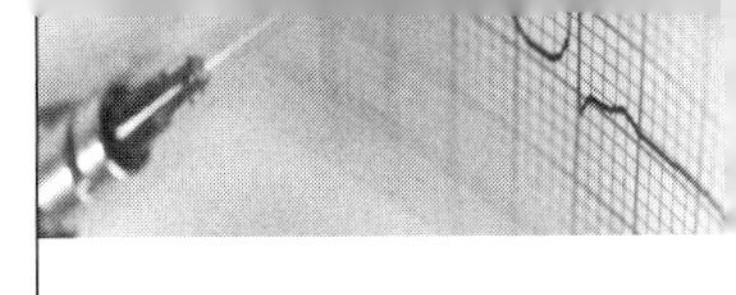

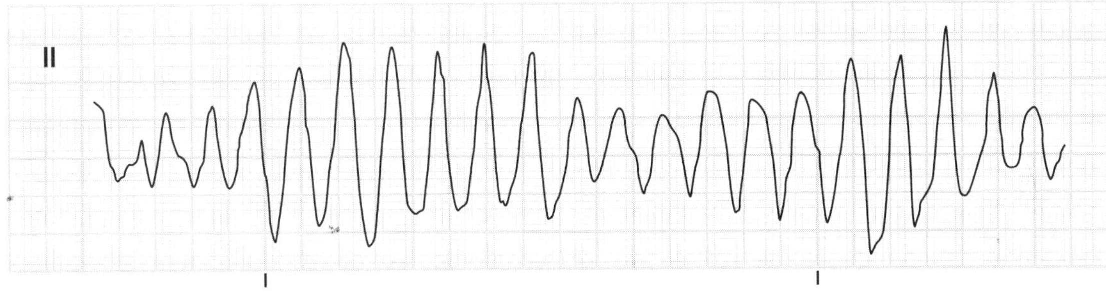

Figure 1-19: Polymorphic ventricular tachycardia.

Rhythm: Irregular

Rate: 200–250 beats/minute

P waves: None

P-R Interval: None

QRS Complex: Variable, but greater than 0.12 seconds, wide and bizarre

P wave to QRS ratio: None

Origin

Polymorphic ventricular tachycardia (Figure 1-19) has complexes that vary in size, shape, and direction from complex to complex. This arrhythmia typically occurs when the QT interval of the original underlying rhythm becomes prolonged, indicating a severe delay in ventricular repolarization. As the ventricles become irritable, an ectopic ventricular pacemaker overrides atrial activity. A variant of polymorphic ventricular tachycardia is Torsades de Pointes (TdP), which means "twisting of points."

Clinical Significance

Polymorphic ventricular tachycardia has many of the same causes as its monomorphic counterpart; however, it is particularly prone to occur after the administration of quinidine and procainamide, both of which are drugs that prolong the QT interval. Hypomagnesemia (low blood magnesium level) is a very common cause of polymorphic ventricular tachycardia. As with monomorphic ventricular tachycardia, the atria do not contract regularly and adequately fill the ventricles before they contract. This results in a marked reduction in cardiac output. Both monomorphic and polymorphic ventricular tachycardias have a high potential for deteriorating to ventricular fibrillation.

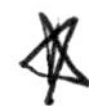

HypoMg = polymorphic V tach

Cardiac Arrest Rhythms

Introduction

This section covers the arrhythmias that do not produce a palpable pulse, leading to cardiac arrest. It is critical that you recognize and treat these rhythms as soon as possible to maximize your patient's chances of survival.

Ventricular Fibrillation/Pulseless Ventricular Tachycardia

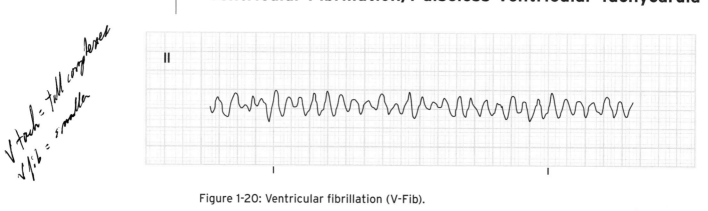

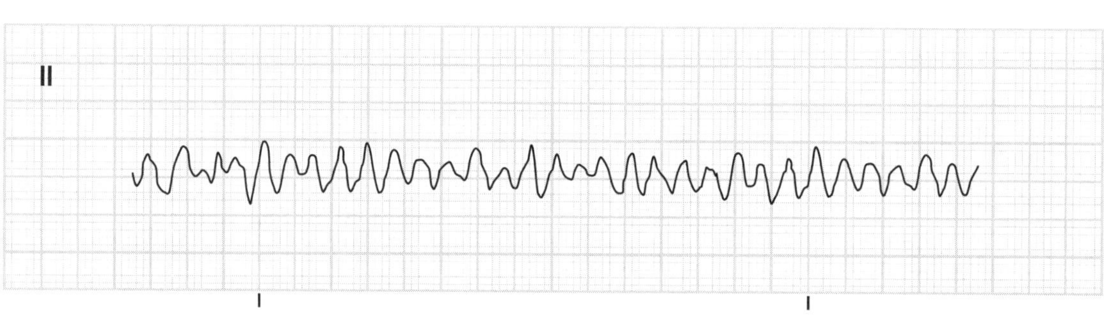

Figure 1-20: Ventricular fibrillation (V-Fib).

Rhythm: Chaotic

Rate: Indeterminate

P waves: None, fibrillatory waves only

P-R Interval: None

QRS Complex: None, fibrillatory waves only

P wave to QRS ratio: None

Origin

Multiple ectopic ventricular pacemakers, which depolarize in a random, chaotic fashion and spread throughout the myocardium, are responsible for ventricular fibrillation.

Clinical Significance

Ventricular fibrillation (Figure 1-20) is a lethal arrhythmia. It is an uncontrolled "quivering" of the myocardium that does not produce a palpable pulse. Ventricular fibrillation is the most common initial rhythm in cardiac arrest. Immediate defibrillation is critical in the management of ventricular fibrillation. Coronary artery disease, which leads to myocardial ischemia or myocardial infarction, is the most common cause of ventricular fibrillation. Other causes include hypoxia, acidosis, and early repolarization of the myocardium (e.g., R on T phenomenon).

Note

Ventricular tachycardia, covered previously in the section on Tachycardia, can present with or without a pulse; therefore, it can occur in patients with cardiac arrest as well. Although not as common as ventricular fibrillation, when it occurs, ventricular tachycardia might be witnessed as the first rhythm before it deteriorates to ventricular fibrillation.

Asystole

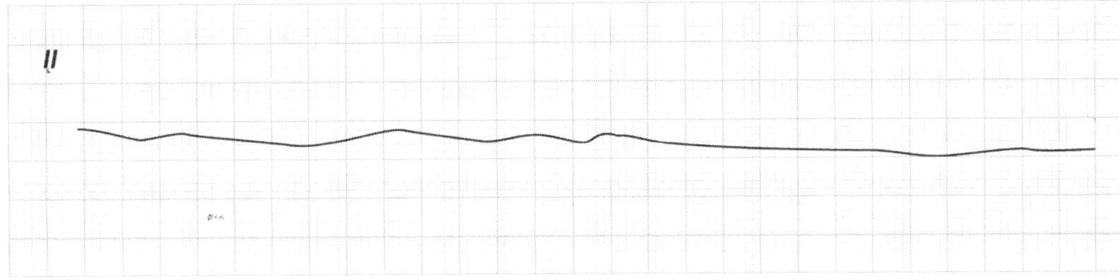

Figure 1-21: Asystole.

Rhythm: None, a flat line

Rate: None

P waves: None

P-R Interval: None

QRS Complex: None

P wave to QRS ratio: None

Origin

In asystole (Figure 1-21), all pacemaker sites in the myocardium fail to generate an electrical impulse. This results in a total absence of electrical and mechanical activity in the myocardium.

Clinical Significance

For obvious reasons, asystole does not produce a pulse. It is commonly the result of untreated ventricular fibrillation. Other causes of asystole include severe hypoxia, acidosis, or electrolyte abnormalities.

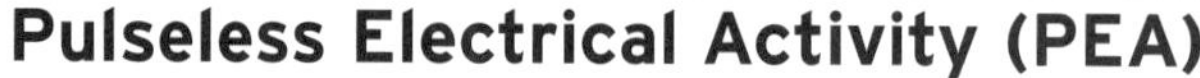

Pulseless Electrical Activity (PEA)

PEA is not a particular cardiac rhythm. Rather, it is a condition in which an organized cardiac rhythm is not accompanied by a palpable pulse. The only organized cardiac rhythm that is not considered to be PEA is pulseless ventricular tachycardia. PEA can be caused by anything that impedes myocardial mechanical activity, although electrical activity resumes. Common causes of PEA include hypoxia, acidosis, pericardial tamponade, tension pneumothorax, and hypovolemia.

Summary

It is important to evaluate the cardiac rhythm of a patient with a cardiac-related chief complaint. Evaluation of the ECG and the patient's signs and symptoms determines the most appropriate treatment approach.

More than one cardiac rhythm can be observed in the same patient. This requires the clinician to be versatile in being able to change the course of management very quickly. It is important to analyze and interpret the patient's cardiac rhythm; however, a careful and systematic assessment is also crucial in determining whether the presenting cardiac rhythm is resulting in hemodynamic compromise.

Management for specific rhythm disturbances is reviewed in Chapter 3 of this study guide.

Chapter 2

Pharmacologic and Electrical Therapy

Introduction

This chapter reviews the most common pharmacologic and electrical interventions used in ACLS to treat patients with a variety of cardiovascular and respiratory system emergencies. After a careful and systematic assessment of your patient, you must determine whether pharmacologic or electrical therapy is indicated.

Although many of the medications reviewed in this chapter have standard adult dosages, alterations in those dosages may be required, depending on the patient's hemodynamic status.

Other medications that may not be listed in this study guide may also be required to treat patients with cardiovascular or respiratory system emergencies.

This chapter reviews the following:

Acute Coronary Syndrome and Stroke
- Aspirin
- Fibrinolytic therapy
- Morphine
- Nitroglycerin
- Oxygen

Antiarrhythmics
- Adenosine
- Amiodarone
- Lidocaine
- Magnesium sulfate
- Procainamide

Calcium Channel Blockers
- Diltiazem
- Verapamil

Electrical Therapy
- Defibrillation
- Synchronized cardioversion
- Transcutaneous pacing

Parasympatholytics
- Atropine

Sympathomimetics
- Epinephrine
- Dopamine
- Vasopressin

Acute Coronary Syndrome and Stroke

Introduction

The medications reviewed in this section, which are used to achieve various therapeutic effects, are indicated in patients who present with signs and symptoms suggestive of an acute coronary syndrome (e.g., myocardial infarction, unstable angina) or acute ischemic stroke.

Aspirin (Acetylsalicylic Acid/ASA)

Therapeutic Effects

- Blocks the formation of thromboxane A_2, thus inhibiting platelet aggregation and vasoconstriction
- Reduces overall mortality from acute myocardial infarction and reduces the incidence of reinfarction and nonfatal stroke

Indications

- Signs and symptoms suggestive of an acute coronary syndrome, such as chest pain or discomfort
- ECG changes that are consistent with acute coronary syndrome, such as ST-segment depression/elevation or T-wave inversion

Contraindications

- Known hypersensitivity to aspirin
- Bleeding disorders (e.g., hemophilia)
- Active ulcer disease or recent gastrointestinal bleeding

Adult Dose

- 2–4 pediatric chewable aspirin (160–325 mg) as soon as possible after the onset of symptoms
  - To achieve a rapid therapeutic blood level, instruct the patient to chew the aspirin before swallowing.

Fibrinolytic Therapy (Thrombolytics)

Therapeutic Effects

- Numerous fibrinolytic agents are on the market, each of which may produce varying mechanisms of action. However, the drugs alteplase (Activase, tPA), anistreplase (Eminase), reteplase (Retavase), streptokinase (Streptase), and tenecteplase (TNKase) produce a similar therapeutic effect, which is the conversion of plasminogen to plasmin. Plasmin destroys the fibrin and fibrinogen matrix of a thrombus (fibrinolysis), thus destroying the clot that is obstructing an artery and reestablishing distal blood flow.

Indications

- Acute myocardial infarction in adults
  - ST-segment elevation of greater than or equal to 1 mm in 2 or more contiguous leads
  - In the context of signs and symptoms of acute myocardial infarction (e.g., chest pain) of no greater than 12 hours duration
- Acute ischemic stroke *(Alteplase is the only fibrinolytic agent approved for use.)*
  - Sudden onset of focal neurologic deficit (e.g., slurred speech, facial droop) or alterations in mental status
  - Absence of intracerebral/subarachnoid hemorrhage (ruled out with head computed tomography [CT])
  - Signs and symptoms not rapidly improving (e.g., transient ischemic attack)
  - Signs and symptoms of no greater than 3 hours duration

Contraindications

- Active internal bleeding within 21 days (menses excluded)
- History of cerebrovascular, intracranial, or intraspinal event within 3 months
  - Stroke
  - Arteriovenous (AV) malformation
  - Neoplasm (tumor)
  - Aneurysm
  - Trauma or surgery
- Major surgery or trauma within 14 days
- Aortic dissection
- Severe uncontrolled hypertension
- Known bleeding disorders (e.g., hemophilia)
- History of prolonged cardiopulmonary resuscitation (CPR) with evidence of thoracic trauma
- Lumbar puncture within 7 days
- Recent arterial puncture at a noncompressible site
- Aspirin or heparin administered within the first 24 hours after acute ischemic stroke

Adult Dose

- Variable, depending on the fibrinolytic agent used

Morphine Sulfate (MSO_4)

Therapeutic Effects

- Morphine is a narcotic analgesic that promotes, through its vasodilatory effects, systemic venous pooling of blood, which reduces venous return to the heart (preload) as well as systemic vascular resistance (afterload). By this mechanism, morphine is effective in reducing myocardial oxygen demand and consumption. Additionally, its narcotic effect reduces chest pain and anxiety.

Indications

- Chest pain in acute coronary syndrome that is not completely relieved by nitroglycerin.
- Cardiogenic pulmonary edema (with a systolic blood pressure greater than 90 mm Hg)

Contraindications

- Hypersensitivity to morphine or other opiate drugs

- Signs of central nervous system depression (e.g., respiratory depression, bradycardia, hypotension)

Adult Dose

- 2 to 4 mg increments via slow IV push given over 1–5 minutes. The dose may be repeated every 5–30 minutes as needed to achieve the desired effect.

  - Should signs of central nervous system (CNS) depression occur, naloxone (Narcan) should be given in a dose of 0.4 to 2 mg via IV or IM push to reverse this effect.

Nitroglycerin (NTG)

Therapeutic Effects

- Nitroglycerin, which is a nitrate, is a smooth muscle relaxant that produces systemic venous pooling of blood through its vasodilatory effects. This effect decreases venous return to the heart (preload) as well as systemic vascular resistance (afterload), resulting in decreased myocardial oxygen consumption.

Indications

- Chest pain suspected to be of cardiac origin
- Cardiogenic pulmonary edema secondary to left-sided congestive heart failure

Contraindications

- Systolic blood pressure of less than 90 mm Hg or greater than 30 mm Hg below baseline
- Severe bradycardia (< 50 beats/min) or tachycardia (> 100 beats/min)
- Use of sildenafil (Viagra) or vardenafil (Levitra) within the past 24 hours; use of tadalafil (Cialis) within the past 48 hours

Adult Dose

- Sublingual tablets: 0.3 or 0.4 mg (1 tablet) repeated in 5-minute intervals to a maximum of three tablets
- Sublingual spray: 1 spray (0.4 mg metered dose) repeated in 5-minute intervals to a maximum of three sprays
- IV infusion: 10–20 mcg/min titrated to desired effect
  - Frequently monitor blood pressure (BP)

Oxygen (O_2)

Therapeutic Effects

- Increases hemoglobin saturation and enhances tissue oxygenation, provided that adequate ventilation and circulation are maintained
- Increases oxygen surface tension in the blood

Indications

- Any suspected cardiovascular, cerebrovascular, or respiratory system emergency
  - Chest pain
  - Altered mental status
  - Shortness of breath
  - Any patient that you think needs it

Contraindications

- None, when given in emergency situations

Dose and Method of Administration (regardless of age)

- Mild hypoxia with *adequate* breathing
  - Nasal cannula at 4 L/min
- Severe hypoxia with *adequate* breathing
  - Nonrebreathing mask at 15 L/min
- Inadequate breathing or apnea
  - Bag-valve mask with reservoir and supplemental oxygen at 15 L/min

Antiarrhythmics

Introduction

Antiarrhythmic medications are used to treat a variety of cardiac arrhythmias, both supraventricular (narrow complex) and ventricular (wide complex) in origin. The medications reviewed in this section are addressed in eACLS.

Adenosine (Adenocard)

Therapeutic Effects

- Adenosine is a naturally occurring (endogenous) nucleoside that is rapidly metabolized. Adenosine slows the discharge rate of the SA node and slows conduction through the AV node, thus restoring a normal sinus rhythm in supraventricular tachycardias.

Indications

- Narrow QRS complex supraventricular tachycardias (e.g., supraventricular tachycardia [SVT]) to slow the ventricular rate and determine the underlying rhythm

Contraindications

- Toxin-induced tachycardias
- Second- or third-degree atrioventricular (AV) block
- Atrial fibrillation/flutter
- Ventricular (wide QRS complex) tachycardia

Adult Dose

- Initial dose
    - 6 mg rapid (over 1–3 seconds) IV push with extremity elevated, followed by a 20 mL saline flush
- Repeat dose
    - 12 mg via rapid IV push 1–2 minutes after initial dose. 12 mg dose may be repeated 1–2 minutes later.
        - Total cumulative dose: 30 mg

Amiodarone (Cordarone)

Therapeutic Effects

- Amiodarone is a diverse antiarrhythmic drug. It blocks sodium, calcium, and potassium channels and inhibits sympathetic nervous system stimulation. In addition, it suppresses sinoatrial (SA) node discharge, thus slowing the heart rate, and it slows conduction at the AV node. Amiodarone is particularly useful for slowing conduction in the His-Purkinje system and in accessory pathways of patients with Wolff-Parkinson-White (WPW) syndrome.

Indications

- V-Fib and pulseless V-Tach that is refractory to defibrillation
- Polymorphic V-Tach and wide-complex tachycardia of uncertain origin
- Stable V-Tach when cardioversion is unsuccessful
- Adjunct to synchronized cardioversion in supraventricular tachycardias (e.g., atrial tachycardia)

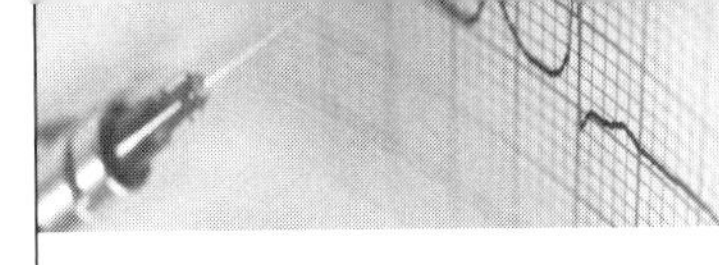

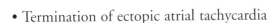

- Termination of ectopic atrial tachycardia
- Rate control in atrial fibrillation and atrial flutter when other therapies prove ineffective

Contraindications

- Known sensitivity to amiodarone
- Sinus node disease with significant bradycardia
- Second- and third-degree AV block

Adult Dose

- V-Fib and pulseless V-Tach
    - 300 mg diluted in 20–30 mL of D_5W via rapid IV push
    - Repeat dose of 150 mg diluted in 20–30 mL of D_5W via rapid IV push 3–5 minutes after the initial dose
- Stable V-Tach, SVT, and atrial flutter/fibrillation
    - 150 mg diluted in 20–30 mL of D_5W via IV push over 10 minutes
        - May repeat this dose every 10 minutes as needed
- 24-hour maintenance infusion
    - 360 mg via IV infusion over the first 6 hours (1.0 mg/min)
    - 540 mg via IV infusion over the remaining 18 hours (0.5 mg/min)
        - Maximum dose: 2.2 grams/24 hours

Lidocaine (Xylocaine)

Therapeutic Effects

- Lidocaine blocks the influx of sodium through the fast channels of the myocardium, which decreases conduction, and therefore irritability, in ischemic areas. This effect increases the V-Fib threshold. Conversely, lidocaine decreases the defibrillation threshold.

Indications

- V-Fib and pulseless V-Tach that is refractory to defibrillation
- Stable wide-complex tachycardias (e.g., V-Tach, wide-complex tachycardias of uncertain origin)

Contraindications

- Known hypersensitivity to lidocaine or "caine" type drugs (e.g., Novocain)
- Sinus bradycardia
- Atrioventricular blocks

Adult Dose

- V-Fib and pulseless V-Tach
    - 1–1.5 mg/kg via rapid IV push
    - Repeat dose of 0.5–0.75 mg/kg every 5–10 minutes for refractory V-Fib and pulseless V-Tach, to a maximum total dose of 3 mg/kg
- Stable V-Tach and wide-complex tachycardia of uncertain origin
    - 1–1.5 mg/kg via rapid IV push
    - Repeat dose of 0.5–0.75 mg/kg every 5–10 minutes to a maximum total dose of 3 mg/kg
- Maintenance infusion
    - 1–4 mg/min titrated to desired effect

Magnesium Sulfate ($MgSO_4$)

Therapeutic Effects

- Officially classified as an electrolyte, magnesium possesses antiarrhythmic-like properties. Magnesium slows the impulse rate of the SA node and suppresses automaticity in partially depolarized cells. In addition, at increased levels, magnesium has CNS depressant properties.

Indications

- Torsades de Pointes (TdP) with a pulse
- Cardiac arrest *only* if Torsades de Pointes *or* suspected hypomagnesemia is present
- Ventricular arrhythmias due to digitalis toxicity

Contraindications

- CNS depression
- Hypermagnesemia
- Hypocalcemia

Adult Dose

- Torsades de Pointes (TdP) with a pulse
    - Loading dose of 1–2 g mixed in 50–100 mL of D_5W, given IV over 5–60 minutes
    - Follow with 0.5–1 g/hour IV, titrated to control Torsades de Pointes
- Cardiac arrest (from hypomagnesemia or Torsades de Pointes)
    - 1–2 g (2–4 mL of a 50% solution) diluted in 10 mL of D_5W, given IV over 5–20 minutes

Procainamide (Pronestyl)

Therapeutic Effects

- Procainamide slows conduction in the atria, ventricles, and His-Purkinje system by prolonging the P-R and Q-T intervals and the refractory period of the AV node. Procainamide slows the refractory period within the atria.

Indications

- Recurrent V-Fib or pulseless V-Tach
- Stable SVT that is uncontrolled with vagal maneuvers or adenosine
- Stable wide-complex tachycardias of uncertain origin
- Atrial fibrillation with rapid ventricular rate in patients with WPW

Contraindications

- Known sensitivity to procainamide or similar medications
- Third-degree AV block (without an artificial pacemaker)
- Digitalis toxicity (may exacerbate AV conduction depression)
- Pre-existing prolongation of the QRS complex and Q-T intervals

Adult Dose

- Recurrent V-Fib and pulseless V-Tach
  - 20 mg/min via IV infusion
  - In urgent situations, up to 50 mg/min may be administered
    - Use of procainamide in cardiac arrest is limited by need for slow infusion and uncertain efficacy
- SVT, atrial fibrillation, and wide-complex tachycardia of uncertain origin
  - 20 mg/min via IV infusion
- Maintenance infusion
  - 1–4 mg/min titrated to desired effect
- Stop procainamide infusion when at least **one** of the following occurs:
  - Arrhythmia suppression
  - Hypotension develops
  - QRS complex widens by greater than 50% of its pretreatment width
  - Maximum dose of 17 mg/kg has been given

Calcium Channel Blockers

Introduction

Calcium channel blockers are used in the treatment of stable narrow-complex tachycardias as well as for rate control in atrial fibrillation and atrial flutter.

Diltiazem (Cardizem)

Therapeutic Effects

- Blocks the movement of calcium ions across the cell membranes of the myocardium and smooth muscles of the vasculature. This effect results in decreased myocardial contractility (negative inotropy), slowing of conduction through the AV node (negative dromotropy), and dilation of the coronary arteries and peripheral vasculature, which decreases myocardial oxygen demand.

Indications

- Control of ventricular rate in atrial fibrillation and atrial flutter
- Adjunct to adenosine to treat stable narrow-complex tachycardias

Contraindications

- Wide-complex tachycardias of uncertain origin
- Poison- or drug-induced tachycardias
- Rapid atrial fibrillation and atrial flutter in patients with WPW
- Sinus node disease
- AV block (without an artificial pacemaker)
- Concurrent administration of beta-blocking drugs (e.g., atenolol, Inderal)
  - May precipitate significant hypotension

Adult Dose

- IV bolus
  - 15–20 mg (0.25 mg/kg) IV over 2 minutes
    - May repeat 15 minutes later at 20–25 mg (0.35 mg/kg) over 2 minutes
- Maintenance infusion
  - 5–15 mg/hour titrated to desired heart rate

Verapamil (Calan, Isoptin)

Therapeutic Effects

- Blocks the movement of calcium ions across the cell membranes of the myocardium and the smooth muscles of the vasculature. This effect results in decreased myocardial contractility (negative inotropy), slowing of conduction

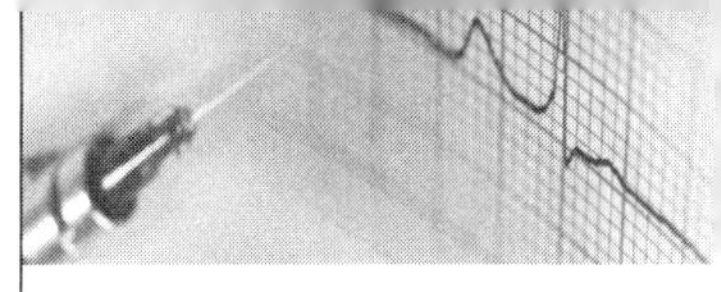

through the AV node (negative dromotropy), and dilation of the coronary arteries and peripheral vasculature, which decreases myocardial oxygen demand.

Indications

- Control of ventricular rate in atrial fibrillation, atrial flutter, and ectopic atrial tachycardia
- Adjunct to adenosine to treat stable narrow-complex tachycardias

Contraindications

- Wide-complex tachycardias of uncertain origin
- Poison- or drug-induced tachycardias
- Rapid atrial fibrillation and atrial flutter in patients with WPW
- Sinus node disease
- AV block (without an artificial pacemaker)
- Concurrent administration of beta-blocking drugs (e.g., atenolol, Inderal)
    - May precipitate significant hypotension

Adult Dose

- 2.5–5 mg via IV push over 2 minutes
    - Repeat dose at 5–10 mg via IV push every 15–30 minutes
        - Maximum dose of 20 mg
- Alternative dosing regimen
    - 5 mg via IV push every 15 minutes
        - Maximum dose of 30 mg

Electrical Therapy

Introduction

Electrical therapy is frequently used in emergency cardiac care for patients who have serious signs and symptoms as a result of their cardiac rhythm. Patients whose heart rates are too slow, too fast, or chaotic and without a pulse need prompt electrical therapy to stabilize their condition.

Defibrillation

Therapeutic Effects

- Defibrillation is the unsynchronized delivery of energy into the myocardium. The therapeutic effect of defibrillation is to stop chaotic electrical activity by literally freezing the heart in animation, so that an organized cardiac pacemaker (e.g., SA or AV node) can dominate and restore a perfusing rhythm.

Indications

- V-Fib and pulseless V-Tach
- Unstable polymorphic V-Tach

Contraindications

- Asystole
  - Routine defibrillation of asystole is not recommended, because it may result in failure to identify and treat the underlying cause of asystole.
- Regular cardiac rhythms with a pulse
- Other health care providers being in physical contact with the patient
  - You must ensure that **no one** is in physical contact with the patient before you perform defibrillation.

Adult Energy Settings[a]

- V-Fib and pulseless V-Tach
  - 360 J (or biphasic equivalent[b]) for first and subsequent shocks
  - Follow each shock *immediately* with CPR
    - Reassess rhythm after 2 minutes of CPR
  - If first defibrillation fails to convert V-Fib or pulseless V-Tach, defibrillate one time, as needed, after every 2 minutes of CPR
- Unstable polymorphic V-Tach
  - 360 J (or biphasic equivalent), repeated as needed
  - Be prepared to perform CPR if patient becomes pulseless

Synchronized Cardioversion

Therapeutic Effects

- Synchronized cardioversion is the timed delivery of energy into the myocardium to correct rapid, regular cardiac rhythms in patients who are unstable as a result of the cardiac rhythm. An internal "synchronizer" times the shock to deliver when it senses an R wave. This avoids delivering the shock during the relative refractory period (down slope of the T wave), which may precipitate V-Fib.

Indications

- Perfusing narrow and wide QRS complex tachycardias (rate ≥ 150 per minute)

---

[a] *If cardiac arrest is unwitnessed, perform 5 cycles (about 2 minutes) of CPR before attempting defibrillation.*

[b] *Biphasic defibrillators shock at lower energy levels (120–150 J). Initial and repeat shocks at biphasic levels are acceptable if they are clinically equivalent to monophasic defibrillation.*

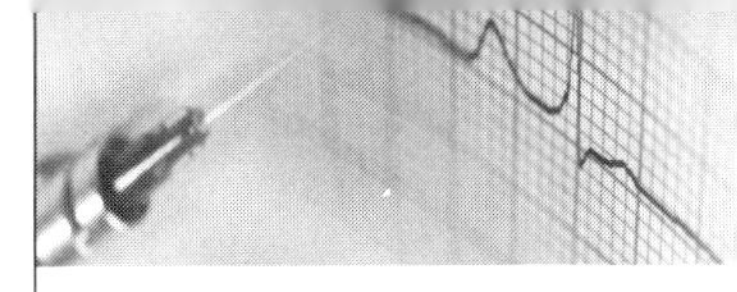

with serious signs and symptoms linked to the tachycardia.

- Monomorphic V-Tach, SVT, atrial fibrillation, atrial flutter

Contraindications

- V-Fib or pulseless V-Tach (requires defibrillation)
- Poison- or drug-induced tachycardia
  - Treat the underlying problem with an antidote, if available.
  - The serious signs and symptoms are related to the poison or drug, not the tachycardia.
- Other health care providers being in physical contact with the patient.
  - You must ensure that **no one** is in physical contact with the patient before you perform synchronized cardioversion.

Adult Energy Settings[c]

- Monomorphic V-Tach and atrial fibrillation
  - Start with 100 J (or biphasic equivalent[d]). Repeat at 200, 300, and 360 J, respectively, if the rhythm is not corrected.
- SVT and atrial flutter
  - Start with 50 J (or biphasic equivalent). Repeat at 100, 200, 300, and 360 J, respectively, if the rhythm is not corrected.

Transcutaneous Cardiac Pacing (TCP)

Therapeutic Effects

- TCP involves using an artificial electrical impulse to increase the electrical discharge rate of a slow, inherent pacemaker in the heart. TCP is the preferred initial cardiac pacing method in emergency cardiac care because it can be initiated quickly and is relatively safe.

Indications

- Symptomatic bradycardia when the patient's signs and symptoms are linked to the bradycardia and atropine is either unavailable or unsuccessful. Examples of cardiac rhythms that may require TCP include:
  - AV blocks (especially second-degree type II and third-degree)
  - Bradycardia with ventricular escape complexes

---

[c] *Sedate the conscious and the semiconscious patient with a benzodiazepine (e.g., Valium, Versed) before performing cardioversion.*

[d] *Biphasic cardioversion, using lower energy levels, is acceptable if it is documented to be clinically equivalent to monophasic cardioversion.*

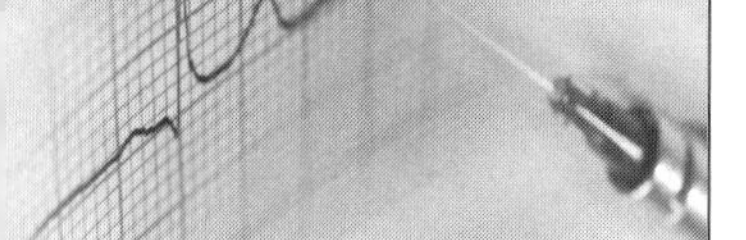

Contraindications

- Severe hypothermia
- Prolonged bradyasystolic cardiac arrest

Adult Energy Settings

- Set pacing rate at 80 bpm.
    - Symptomatic bradycardia
        - Increase output (mA) from the minimum setting until consistent electrical capture is achieved, as evidenced by a widening of the QRS complex and a broad T wave after each pacer spike.
        - Increase 2 mA further for a safety margin.

Parasympatholytics

Introduction

Also referred to as parasympathetic blockers, vagolytic, and anticholinergic drugs, parasympatholytics block the parasympathetic nervous system via the vagus nerve and are used to treat symptomatic bradycardias (absolute and relative) caused by increased vagal tone.

Atropine Sulfate

Therapeutic Effects

- By blocking the effects of the parasympathetic nervous system (e.g., vagus nerve), atropine increases the heart rate because it accelerates the discharge rate of the SA node. Atropine also enhances conduction through the atria and the AV node.

Indications

- Symptomatic bradycardia (absolute or relative)
- Asystole
- Bradycardic pulseless electrical activity (PEA)

Contraindications

- Glaucoma (atropine causes pupillary dilation)
- Atropine may not be effective in treating bradycardia accompanied by second-degree type II and third-degree AV blocks.
- Tachycardia
- Denervated hearts (e.g., heart transplant patients). Proceed with TCP or catecholamines instead.

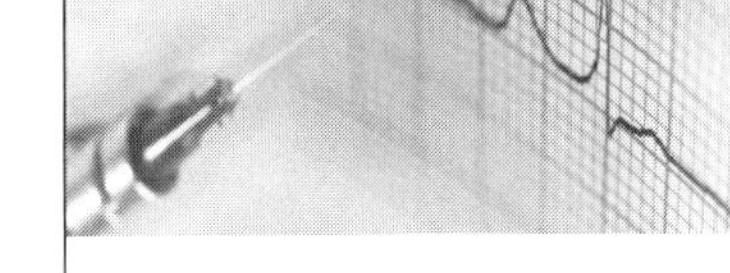

Adult Dose[e]

- Symptomatic bradycardia
  - 0.5 mg via rapid IV push
    - Repeat every 3–5 minutes to a maximum dose of 3 mg.
    - Must give rapidly. Atropine will cause a paradoxical bradycardia if it is given too slowly.
- Asystole and bradycardic PEA
  - 1 mg via rapid IV push
    - Repeat every 3–5 minutes to a maximum dose of 3 mg.

Sympathomimetics

Introduction

Sympathomimetic drugs mimic the effects of the sympathetic nervous system and are thus used to increase the heart rate and blood pressure. Drugs in this category are usually the synthetically produced equivalent to what is endogenous (naturally occurring) in the human body.

Epinephrine (Adrenalin)

Therapeutic Effects

- Epinephrine is a naturally occurring catecholamine. It possesses positive alpha and beta adrenergic effects. Its alpha effects result in vasoconstriction, thus increasing the blood pressure. Its selective $beta_1$ effects result in increased heart rate (positive chronotropy), and increased myocardial contractility (positive inotropy). Its selective $beta_2$ effects cause relaxation of bronchial smooth muscle (bronchodilation).

Indications

- Cardiac arrest
  - V-Fib/pulseless V-Tach, asystole, PEA
- Symptomatic bradycardia
  - After atropine and pacing
- Severe hypotension
  - Treat with fluid boluses first.
- Anaphylactic shock
  - Combined with fluid boluses, corticosteroids, and antihistamines

---

[e] *Give 2–2.5 mg diluted in 10 mL of normal saline if given ET.*

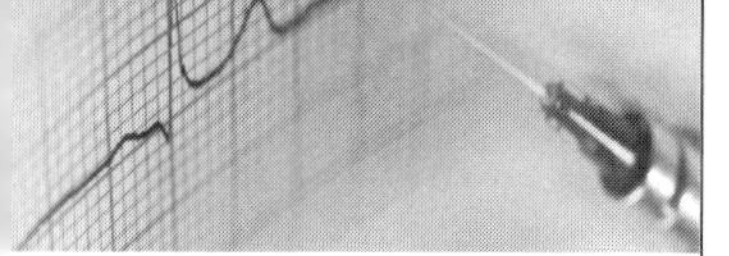

Contraindications

- Tachycardia
- Hypertension
- Do not mix with alkaline solutions (e.g., sodium bicarbonate), because deactivation of epinephrine, as with all catecholamines, will occur.

Adult Dose[f]

- Cardiac arrest
    - 1 mg (10 mL of 1:10,000 solution) every 3–5 minutes, followed by a 20 mL flush of normal saline
    - There is no maximum dose of epinephrine when it is given for persistent cardiac arrest.
- Symptomatic bradycardia or severe hypotension
    - 2–10 mcg/min
        - Add 1 mg of epinephrine (1 mL of 1:1,000 solution) to 500 mL of normal saline and infuse at 1–5 mL/min.

Dopamine (Intropin)

Therapeutic Effects

- Dopamine is a naturally occurring catecholamine. Its physiologic effects vary with increasing doses. At medium or "cardiac" (5–10 mcg/kg/min) doses, dopamine acts directly on $beta_1$ receptors and causes increased myocardial contractility (increased inotropy) as well as increased SA node discharge and increased heart rate (positive chronotropy). Doses greater than 10 mcg/kg/min (vasopressor dose) stimulate alpha receptors, resulting in an increase in systemic vascular resistance (vasoconstriction). The dosing range of dopamine depends on the patient's clinical condition.

Indications

- Symptomatic bradycardia
    - After atropine, pacing, and epinephrine
- Hypotension (systolic BP $\leq$ 70–100 mm Hg) with signs and symptoms of shock
    - Consider fluid boluses first because dopamine should never be given on an empty tank.

Contraindications

- Known hypersensitivity to dopamine
- Hypovolemia

---

f Give 2–2.5 mg diluted in 10 mL of normal saline if given ET.

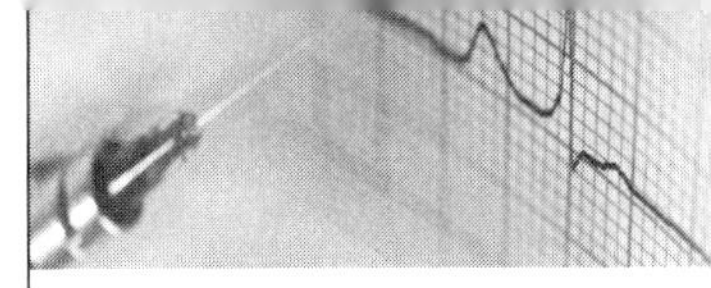

- Tachydysrhythmias or V-Fib
- Pheochromocytoma (an adrenal tumor that produces epinephrine)
- Concurrent use of monoamine oxidase (MAO) inhibitors (e.g., Marplan, Parnate, Nardil)
- Do not mix with alkaline solutions (e.g., sodium bicarbonate), because deactivation of dopamine, as with all catecholamines, will occur.

Adult Dose

- As an IV infusion, mix 400–800 mg of dopamine in 250 mL of normal saline, D_5W, or lactated Ringer's solution, and titrate based on the patient's clinical response:
  - Symptomatic bradycardia
    - 2–10 mcg/kg/min
  - Profound hypotension (nonhypovolemic)
    - 10–20 mcg/kg/min

Vasopressin (Pitressin Synthetic)

Therapeutic Effects

- Vasopressin is an antidiuretic hormone (ADH) that is produced in the pituitary gland in the brain. Vasopressin binds to specific receptors, specifically vasopressin (V) receptors. There are two types of V receptors, V_1 (V_1a and V_1b) and V_2. V_1a receptor stimulation produces potent vasoconstriction, whereas V_2 receptor stimulation produces vasodilation. Compared with epinephrine, vasopressin possesses a greater vasoconstrictive effect, especially in an acidotic and hypoxic environment (e.g., cardiac arrest). In addition, vasopressin does not increase myocardial oxygen consumption.

Indications

- Used to replace the first or second dose of epinephrine for patients in cardiac arrest from V-Fib/pulseless V-Tach, asystole, and PEA

Contraindications

- Known sensitivity to vasopressin
- Acute coronary syndrome
  - Vasopressin may exacerbate hypertension because of its vasoconstrictive effects.

Adult Dose

- 40 units via IV push as a *one-time dose*
  - Wait approximately 10 minutes after vasopressin administration before initiating/resuming epinephrine therapy.

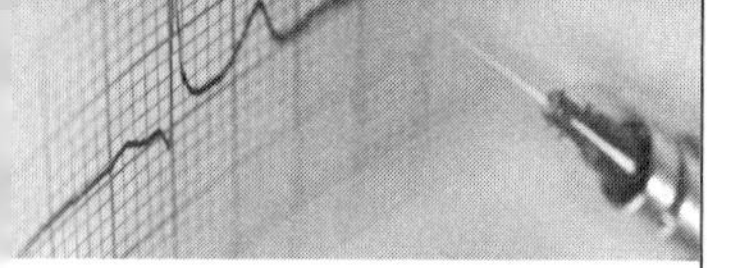

Summary

Selecting the most appropriate emergency intervention for your patient (pharmacologic or electrical) depends on a careful and systematic assessment in order to determine whether the patient is unstable, as evidenced by serious signs and symptoms (e.g., chest pain, altered mental state, shortness of breath). If the patient is unstable, you must determine whether the cardiac rhythm is causing the patient's signs and symptoms or the result of an underlying condition.

When you are preparing to administer a medication, it is important to remember the "six rights" of medication administration, which are:

- **Right** patient
- **Right** drug
- **Right** time
- **Right** dose
- **Right** route
- **Right** documentation

Medication doses and routes may vary, depending on the patient's condition. A particular dose and route for a medication may be therapeutic for one condition but may be detrimental for another.

Chapter 3

Patient Assessment and eACLS Case Review

Introduction

The first part of this chapter reviews the general assessment and treatment of patients who are not in cardiac arrest, as well as of patients who are in cardiac arrest. The second part reviews the 10 cases addressed in the eACLS program.

ACLS often provides a *general approach to treatment.* Additional treatment or variations in treatment may be required, depending on the patient's clinical condition and clinical response to your interventions.

This chapter reviews the following:

Assessment and Treatment of Non–Cardiac Arrest Patients

- Assessing the patient for serious signs and symptoms
- Providing universal treatment for the non-cardiac arrest patient

Assessment and Treatment of Cardiac Arrest Patients

- Assessing the patient for underlying causes of cardiac arrest
- Providing universal treatment for the cardiac arrest patient
- Post–cardiac arrest resuscitation management

eACLS Case Review

- Case 1: Acute coronary syndromes (ACS)
- Case 2: Asystole
- Case 3: Automated external defibrillation (AED)
- Case 4: Bradycardia
- Case 5: Narrow-complex tachycardia
- Case 6: Pulseless electrical activity (PEA)
- Case 7: Respiratory arrest
- Case 8: Stroke
- Case 9: Ventricular fibrillation
- Case 10: Wide-complex tachycardia

Assessment and Treatment of Non–Cardiac Arrest Patients

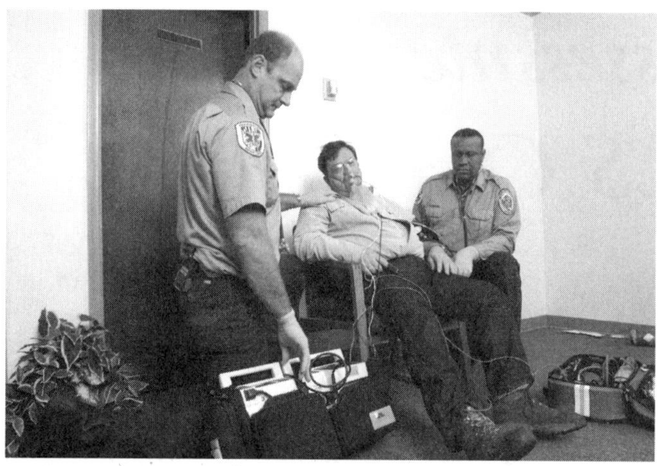

Introduction

Successful management of a conscious patient experiencing a cardiovascular or respiratory system emergency requires a careful and systematic assessment of the patient and selection of the appropriate treatment algorithm.

This section reviews the basic assessment and treatment principles specific to patients who are not in cardiac arrest.

Assessing the Patient for Serious Signs and Symptoms

To prevent cardiac arrest in your patient, you must perform a careful and systematic assessment aimed at identifying serious signs and symptoms linked to their condition or cardiac rhythm (Table 3-1). The presence of serious signs and symptoms indicates that your patient is hemodynamically unstable and requires treatment that differs from that of the stable patient.

Table 3-1: Serious Signs and Symptoms

- Serious signs
  - Altered mental status
  - Pulmonary edema
  - Jugular venous distention
- Serious symptoms
  - Chest pain or pressure
  - Shortness of breath
  - Dyspnea on exertion

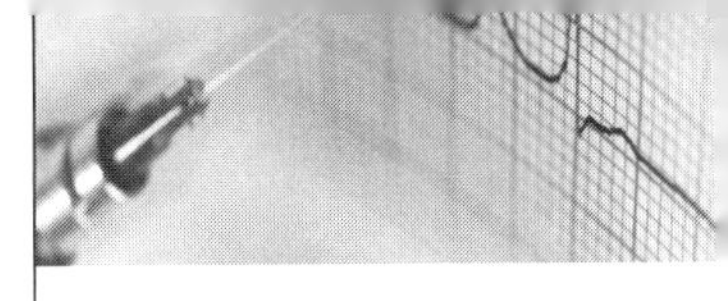

Universal Treatment for the Non-Cardiac Arrest Patient

Certain interventions must be performed on all non–cardiac arrest patients who present with a cardiovascular or respiratory system emergency, regardless of their presenting cardiac rhythm. Table 3-2 reviews those interventions as well as the reason(s) that they are performed.

Table 3-2: Universal Treatment for the Non-Cardiac Arrest Patient

- Supplemental oxygen
    - Supplemental oxygen is the first drug administered to spontaneously breathing patients with a cardiovascular or respiratory system emergency.
        - Nasal cannula at 2–4 L/min for patients without significant hypoxia
        - Nonrebreathing mask at 15 L/min for patients with significant hypoxia
        - Positive-pressure ventilatory support for inadequately breathing patients
- Pulse oximetry
    - The pulse oximeter indicates gross abnormalities, not subtle changes.
    - Administer oxygen in a concentration that maintains oxygen saturations (SpO_2) of greater than 90%.
- Cardiac monitoring
    - Cardiac monitoring is an essential assessment tool that is used to identify potentially life-threatening cardiac dysrhythmias.
    - If available, a 12-lead ECG should be obtained to gather additional information regarding your patient's condition.
- Intravenous therapy
    - IV therapy is necessary in order to administer medications to treat the patient's condition or to give fluid boluses if the patient's blood pressure is low.

Summary

Treating a patient who is not in cardiac arrest but has a cardiovascular or respiratory system emergency requires a careful and systematic assessment to determine whether the patient is stable or unstable. Your assessment findings will enable you to select the most appropriate treatment for the patient's specific condition.

All patients with a cardiovascular or respiratory system emergency require supplemental oxygen, cardiac monitoring, and intravenous therapy. The goal in managing the conscious patient is to prevent cardiac arrest.

Assessment and Treatment of Cardiac Arrest Patients

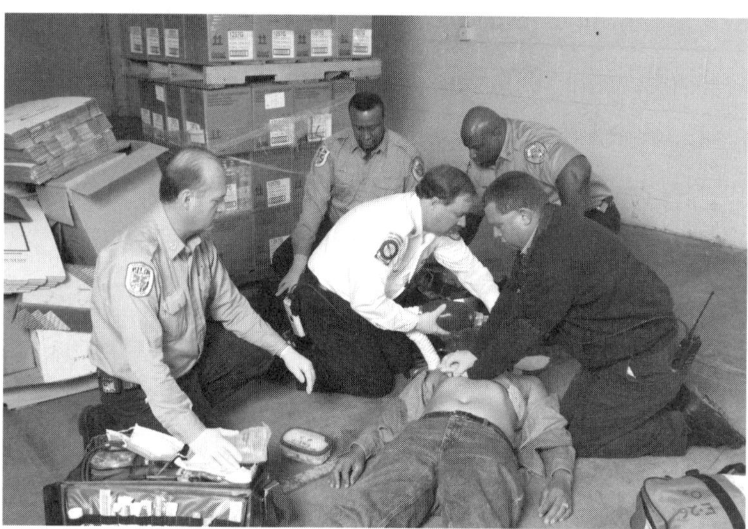

Introduction

Successful management of a patient in cardiac arrest requires a careful and systematic assessment, immediate identification of their cardiac rhythm, and selection of the appropriate treatment algorithm.

This section reviews the basic assessment and treatment principles specific to patients who are in cardiac arrest.

Assessing the Patient for Underlying Causes of Cardiac Arrest

Without carefully assessing the patient, including past medical history and events that preceded the cardiac arrest, a potentially reversible underlying cause that is directly linked to the cardiac arrest may be missed. This means that therapies such as defibrillation and epinephrine and other pharmacologic agents would be of minimal or no benefit until the underlying cause can be identified and corrected.

Table 3-3 summarizes the common causes of cardiac arrest, clinical findings suggestive of each cause, and the specific treatment aimed at reversing each cause. The mnemonic "6 Hs and 6 Ts" will help you remember the potentially reversible underlying causes of cardiac arrest. You should evaluate any patient in cardiac arrest for a potentially reversible cause.

Table 3-3: Underlying Causes of Cardiac Arrest (6 Hs and 6 Ts)

- **H**ypovolemia
  - History of trauma or severe dehydration, flat jugular veins; ECG is rapid with narrow QRS complexes.
    - Give 500 mL bolus of normal saline, and then reassess.
- **H**ypoxia
  - Profound cyanosis, suggestive blood gas readings, airway problems; ECG rhythm is slow.
    - Ensure effective oxygenation and ventilation.
- **H**ydrogen ion (acidosis)
  - History of diabetes (e.g., hyperglycemic ketoacidosis), suggestive blood gas readings, bicarbonate-responsive preexisting acidosis, renal failure, or smaller-amplitude QRS complexes
    - Ensure effective oxygenation and ventilation *first,* then consider sodium bicarbonate
- **H**yperkalemia/hypokalemia
  - History of renal failure, recent dialysis, diuretic use, and abnormal ECG findings (e.g., tall, peaked T waves, flattened T waves, wide QRS, QT prolongation)
    - Calcium chloride or sodium bicarbonate for hyperkalemia
    - Rapid but controlled infusion of potassium and magnesium for hypokalemia
- **H**ypothermia
  - History of recent exposure to cold environment, low core body temperature
    - Remove from cold environment
    - Perform active internal rewarming
    - Limit defibrillations to one attempt and withhold cardiac medications until core body temperature is raised above 86°F (30°C).
- **H**ypoglycemia
  - Diabetic with history of insulin overdose (intentional or accidental), blood glucose level less than 70 mg/dL
    - 25 g (50 mL) of 50% dextrose (D_{50})
- **T**ablets (intentional/accidental overdose [OD])
  - History of ingestion, empty bottles at scene, abnormal neurologic exam, bradycardia, tachycardia, prolonged QT interval
    - Intubation, gastric lavage, Narcan (narcotics), sodium bicarbonate (tricyclic antidepressants), other antidotes specific to ingestion

Continued

Table 3-3 Continued

- Tamponade (cardiac)
  - ▫ History of thoracic trauma, pulse not palpable during CPR, jugular venous distention; ECG rhythm is rapid with narrow QRS complexes.
    - Pericardiocentesis
- Tension pneumothorax
  - ▫ History of thoracic trauma, pulse not palpable during CPR, jugular venous distention, absent breath sounds on the affected side, decreased compliance when ventilating, and contralateral tracheal shift (late)
    - Needle decompression (thoracentesis)
- Thrombosis (coronary, ACS)
  - ▫ History suggestive of acute myocardial infarction (AMI), ST-segment and T-wave changes
    - Fibrinolytics
- Thrombosis (pulmonary)
  - ▫ Sudden onset of dyspnea, pleuritic chest pain, and cyanosis before arrest, pulse not palpable during CPR, jugular venous distention
    - Consult with physician
- Trauma
  - ▫ History of multiple systems trauma (e.g., head, chest, abdominal), signs of profound blood loss, signs of increased intracranial pressure, external signs of trauma
    - Treatment that is specific for each injury (i.e., volume replacement, pericardiocentesis, needle thoracentesis, etc.)

Universal Treatment for the Cardiac Arrest Patient

There are certain interventions that must be carried out in *all* cases of cardiac arrest, *regardless* of the presenting cardiac rhythm. Table 3-4 reviews those interventions as well as the reason(s) that they are performed.

Table 3-4: Universal Treatment for the Cardiac Arrest Patient

- **CPR**
  - ▫ *Effective* CPR keeps the heart and brain perfused until the patient's abnormal cardiac rhythm can be corrected with the appropriate treatment.
    - During CPR: push hard and push fast, deliver 100 compressions per minute, allow *full* recoil of the chest in between compressions, and minimize interruptions in CPR (10 seconds or less)

Continued

Table 3-4 Continued

- **Endotracheal intubation**
  - Patients in cardiac arrest are at a high risk for aspiration of stomach contents; therefore, their airway should be secured with an endotracheal tube as soon as possible.
  - Before you perform intubation, the patient's airway must be open and clear of secretions or potential obstructions. A 2- to 3-minute period of preoxygenation with a bag-valve mask or a pocket mask device, both attached to supplemental oxygen, should precede intubation.
- **Vascular Access**
  - Intravenous (IV) or intraosseous (IO) access needs to be established in order to administer cardiac drugs and, if needed, fluid boluses (normal saline or lactated Ringer's). The IV and IO routes have shown to be equally effective with regard to the medication's onset of action.
    - The IV and IO routes are clearly preferred over the endotracheal (ET) route for medication administration. However, in the absence of IV or IO access, certain medications—lidocaine, epinephrine, atropine, and naloxone—may be given down the ET tube. The optimal endotracheal dose of most drugs is unknown, but is typically 2–2.5 times the recommended IV/IO dose.
- **Vasopressors**
  - Epinephrine, 1 mg of a 1:10,000 solution, is administered every 3–5 minutes in patients in cardiac arrest and should continue until return of spontaneous circulation (ROSC) occurs.
    - Vasopressin, in a *one-time dose* of 40 units, may be used to replace the first or second dose of epinephrine
- **Circulation of cardiac drugs**
  - All cardiac drugs must be circulated with *effective* CPR (push hard and push fast) in order to return the drugs to the central circulation.
- **Identify and correct underlying causes.**
  - If a careful assessment of your patient is performed, a potentially reversible cause of the cardiac arrest can be identified and corrected, thus increasing the chances of a successful resuscitation.

Post-Cardiac Arrest Resuscitation Management

If a pulse and perfusing rhythm are successfully restored, you must perform certain interventions to prevent the recurrence of cardiac arrest. If the patient re-arrests, the chances of a second successful resuscitation are much lower. Prevention of recurrent cardiac arrest can be maximized by performing the appropriate postresuscitation management (Table 3-5).

Table 3-5: Post-Cardiac Arrest Resuscitation Management

- Assess the patient's airway.
  - Ensure adequate ventilation.
  - Reassess ET tube placement.
- Assess the patient's blood pressure.
  - If BP is low, consider a 500 mL bolus of normal saline, then reassess.
  - Initiate dopamine infusion if fluids fail to increase BP.
- Antiarrhythmic infusion
  - Required if patient was in V-Fib or pulseless V-Tach and was successfully converted with an antiarrhythmic agent
    - Amiodarone or lidocaine
  - Titrate antiarrhythmic infusions to the desired effect

Summary

When treating a patient in cardiac arrest, you must focus on identifying and correcting the underlying cause of the cardiac arrest. Failure to do so will significantly decrease the likelihood of a successful resuscitation.

Certain interventions must be performed on all patients in cardiac arrest, regardless of their presenting cardiac rhythm. These interventions are aimed at maintaining effective ventilation and circulation until the patient's abnormal cardiac rhythm can be corrected with the appropriate treatment.

The appropriate post-cardiac arrest resuscitation management prevents the patient from redeveloping cardiac arrest. Patients who re-develop cardiac arrest are more difficult to resuscitate a second time.

eACLS Case Review

Introduction

This section reviews the 10 cases addressed in the eACLS program and is intended to provide you with a review of the assessment and management of patients with cardiovascular and respiratory system emergencies.

Remember that a careful and systematic assessment of the patient and selection of the appropriate treatment algorithm are critical aspects of patient care that will maximize the chances of a favorable patient outcome.

eACLS Case 1: Acute Coronary Syndromes (ACS)

Introduction

eACLS Case 1 focuses on the assessment and management of the patient who presents with an acute coronary syndrome (ACS), which is a term used to describe either unstable angina pectoris or acute myocardial infarction (AMI). Most patients with ACS present with chest pain or discomfort. Because the characteristics of the chest pain are the same for both angina and acute MI, the differentiation between the two is often difficult, if not impossible. For this reason, it is best to err on the side of treating the patient with chest pain or discomfort as though an acute MI is in progress.

Signs and Symptoms of Acute Coronary Syndrome

The single most common symptom of an acute coronary syndrome is retrosternal chest pressure. Commonly, the patient will perceive this pressure as discomfort rather than actual pain. This chest pressure or discomfort typically last longer than 15 minutes and is often unrelieved by rest and/or nitroglycerin.

The signs and symptoms of an acute coronary syndrome (Table 3-6) indicate myocardial ischemia. Some patients may present with very few signs and symptoms, whereas others may have many.

Table 3-6: Signs and Symptoms of Acute Coronary Syndrome

- Pressure, squeezing, or discomfort in the center of the chest, generally lasting longer than 15 minutes
  - May radiate to the shoulders, neck, arms, or jaw, or in the back or between the scapulae
- Lightheadedness, nausea, or fainting
- Shortness of breath
  - May occur without provocation or with exertion
- Feeling of impending doom

Immediate Assessment and Management

Within the first 10 minutes after a patient presents with signs and symptoms of an acute coronary syndrome, an immediate assessment must occur, which is aimed at diagnosing the patient's problem and providing the appropriate treatment.

Immediate general treatment for the patient with an ACS, which should occur simultaneously with the assessment, is aimed at ensuring adequate oxygenation and ventilation, and relieving pain. The mnemonic "MONA," which stands for **mor**phine, **o**xygen, **n**itroglycerin, and **a**spirin, will help you recall the immediate treatment interventions for the patient with an ACS. Although MONA does not represent the actual sequence of treatment, it is a useful mnemonic to remember. Table 3-7 summarizes the sequence of immediate assessment and management for the patient with an ACS.

Table 3-7: Immediate Assessment and Management of the Patient with ACS

- Administer supplemental oxygen.
  - Nasal cannula at 1–4 L/min, or nonrebreathing mask at 15 L/min for more severe cases
    - Monitor oxygen saturation and maintain above 90%.
- Administer aspirin, 160–325 mg.
  - To achieve a rapid therapeutic blood level, instruct the patient to chew the aspirin before swallowing it.
  - Aspirin should **not** be given if the patient has a hypersensitivity to salicylates or a known bleeding disorder (e.g., hemophilia).
- Assess vital signs.
- Apply cardiac monitor and obtain 12-lead ECG tracing.
- Initiate IV of normal saline.
  - You should also obtain cardiac serum markers, electrolytes, and coagulation studies, if possible.
- Administer nitroglycerin (NTG) sublingual tablets or spray.
  - Administer up to 3 nitroglycerin tablets or spray, 5 minutes apart.
- Give morphine, 2–4 mg via slow IV push.
  - If three NTG treatments fail to *completely* relieve the patient's chest pain or discomfort, administer morphine sulfate.

Targeted History for Fibrinolytic Therapy

In conjunction with 12-lead ECG findings, and within the first 10 minutes, you should perform a brief, targeted history and physical examination, with the focus being on eligibility for fibrinolytic therapy. If they are administered within 12 hours of the onset of symptoms, fibrinolytic agents, also called "clot busters," can significantly reduce the size of a myocardial infarction, thus preserving cardiac muscle.

Numerous fibrinolytic agents are on the market, and although their individual doses vary, their mechanisms of action are all similar. Common fibrinolytic agents include recombinant alteplase (Activase), also known as tissue plasminogen activator (tPA), anistreplase (Eminase), recombinant retaplase (Retavase), streptokinase (Streptase), and tenecteplase (TNKase).

The indications, or "inclusion criteria," for fibrinolytic therapy (Table 3-8) must be carefully matched to the contraindications, or "exclusion criteria" (Table 3-9), because if they are administered to the wrong patient, fibrinolytic agents can be lethal.

Table 3-8: Inclusion Criteria for Fibrinolytic Therapy

- ST-segment elevation (≥1 mm in ≥ 2 contiguous leads)
- New or presumably new left bundle branch block (LBBB)
  - The first two signs are conclusive *only* with a 12-lead ECG.
- Signs and symptoms of ACS (see Table 3-6)
- Onset of symptoms < 12 hours ago

Figure 3-1 represents a 12-lead ECG tracing that indicates an acute anteroseptal wall myocardial infarction (ST-segment elevation in leads V_1–V_4) in progress. If the patient met the appropriate criteria, he or she would benefit from fibrinolytic therapy. For an in-depth analysis of 12-lead ECGs, refer to the text *12-Lead ECG: The Art of Interpretation* by Tomas B. Garcia, MD, and Neil Holtz, EMT-P (Jones and Bartlett Publishers, 2001).

Other Reperfusion Strategies

Depending on the patient's presentation and hemodynamic status, other reperfusion strategies may be more appropriate for their condition. Such strategies include percutaneous coronary interventions (PCI), such as a coronary angioplasty with or without stent placement, and coronary artery bypass grafting (CABG).

A careful assessment of the patient's history and hemodynamic status determines which reperfusion intervention is most appropriate.

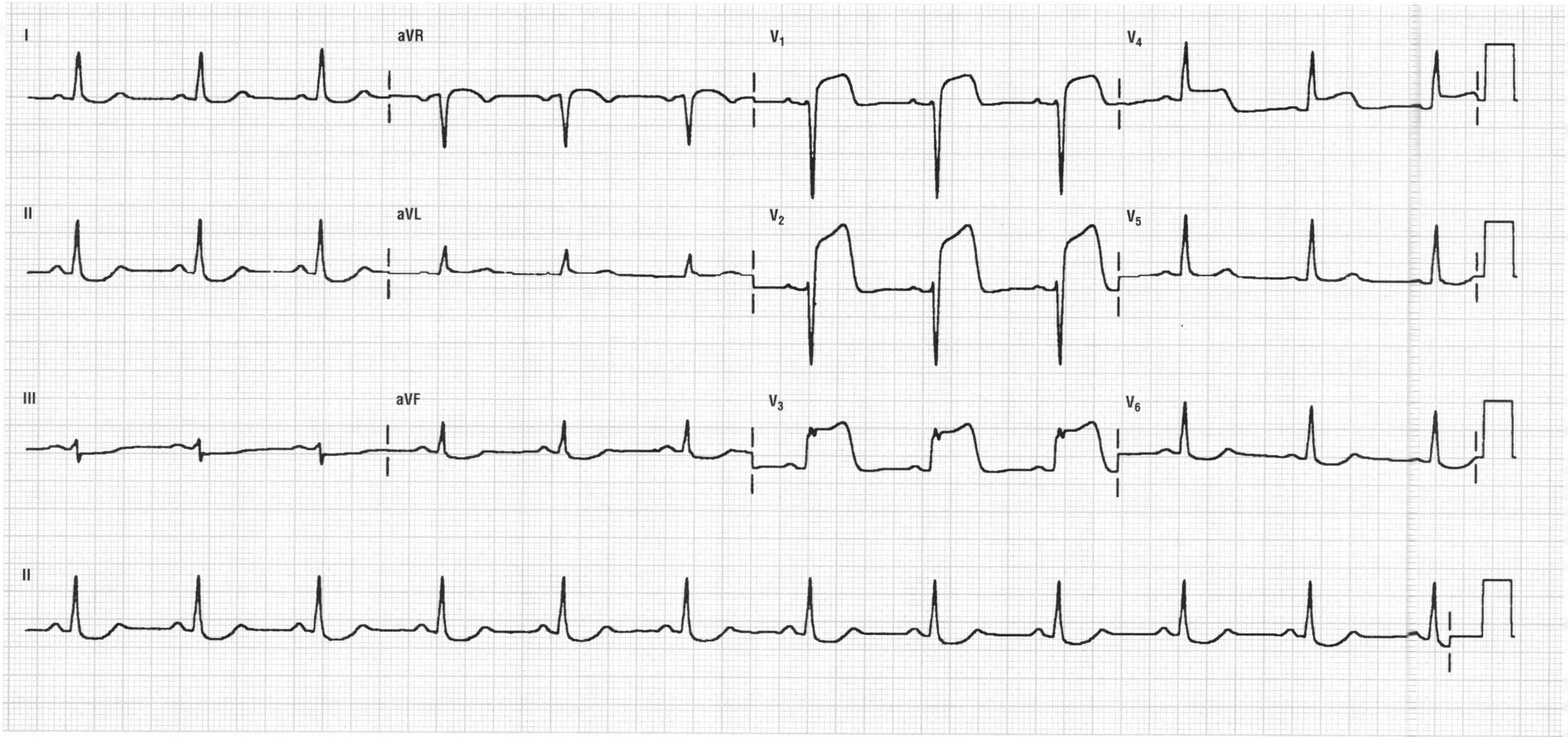

Figure 3-1: Acute anteroseptal wall AMI in progress.

Table 3-9: Exclusion Criteria for Fibrinolytic Therapy

- Active internal bleeding (excluding menses) within the past 21 days
  - History of a cerebrovascular, intracranial, or intraspinal event within the past 3 months
  - Stroke
  - Arteriovenous (AV) malformation
  - Space-occupying intracranial lesion (tumor/neoplasm)
  - Aneurysm
  - Recent trauma or surgery
- Major surgery or serious trauma within the past 14 days
- Aortic dissection
- Severe, uncontrolled hypertension
- Known bleeding disorders (e.g., hemophilia)
- Prolonged CPR with evidence of thoracic trauma
- Lumbar puncture (spinal tap) within the past 7 days
- Recent arterial puncture at a noncompressible site

Summary

The patient who presents with signs and symptoms of an acute coronary syndrome requires an immediate assessment within 10 minutes of presentation. Parameters such as 12-lead electrocardiography, cardiac serum marker analysis, and a brief targeted history with emphasis on potential fibrinolytic candidacy are essential.

Immediate management is aimed at ensuring adequate oxygenation and ventilation and administering pharmacologic interventions to reduce pain and anxiety.

Based on 12-lead ECG findings and a careful assessment of the patient, the most appropriate reperfusion strategy can be selected. The adage "time is muscle" definitely applies and should be remembered when treating the patient with an acute coronary syndrome. If the patient is not assessed and managed within a short period of time, areas of myocardial ischemia or injury will enlarge. This could lead to cardiogenic shock (pump failure), which has a high mortality rate.

eACLS Case 2: Asystole

Introduction

eACLS Case 2 focuses on the assessment and management of the patient in asystole. Asystole represents a total absence of both cardiac electrical and mechanical activity on the cardiac monitor, thus producing a "flat line" (Figure 3-2). Unfortunately, asystole is rarely associated with a positive outcome.

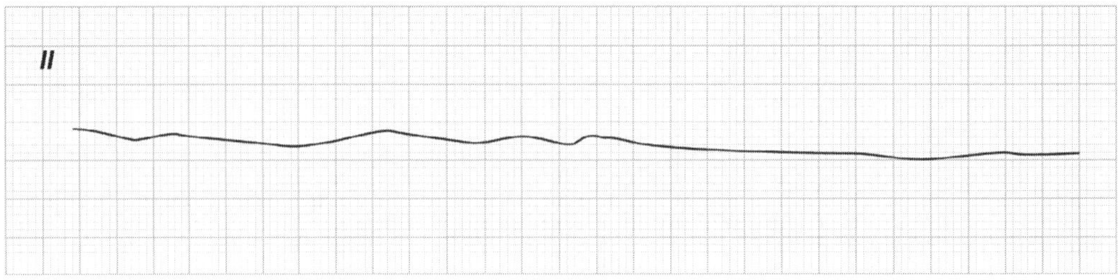

Figure 3-2: Asystole.

Treatment for Asystole

After verification of cardiac arrest and confirmation of asystole, you must assess another lead, because asystole in one lead may actually be fine V-Fib in another. Treatment of the patient (Table 3-10) in asystole requires CPR, airway management, the appropriate medications, and a careful assessment to determine why the patient developed cardiac arrest.

Table 3-10: Treatment for Asystole

- Confirm pulselessness and apnea
  - If the arrest was witnessed, begin CPR and apply a cardiac monitor as soon as it is available
  - If the arrest was not witnessed, perform 5 cycles (about 2 minutes) of CPR, and then apply the cardiac monitor
- Evaluate the cardiac rhythm with defibrillator (quick-look or multi-pads)
  - Confirm asystole
    - Check another lead
    - Increase the gain and sensitivity on the cardiac monitor
  - If fine V-Fib is present, defibrillate at once
- Continue CPR
- Perform endotracheal intubation and establish vascular access (IV or IO)
- Administer epinephrine, 1 mg of a 1:10,000 solution via rapid IV/IO push every 3–5 minutes
  - Vasopressin, in a *one-time dose* of 40 units, can be used to replace the first or second dose of epinephrine

Continued

Table 3-10: continued

- Administer atropine, 1 mg via rapid IV/IO push every 3–5 minutes, to a maximum dose of 3 mg
  - Use shorter dosing intervals (every 3 minutes) for asystolic patients
- Evaluate for and treat the underlying cause of asystole
  - 6 Hs and 6 Ts
- Consider termination of resuscitative efforts
  - The determination to cease resuscitative efforts should be based on the following:
    - Was acceptable basic life support (BLS) continued throughout the arrest?
    - Was an advanced airway device placed and successfully maintained?
    - If present, was V-Fib defibrillated?
    - Was vascular access (e.g., IV or IO) established?
    - Were all rhythm-appropriate drugs administered?
    - Were potentially reversible causes ruled out or corrected?
    - Has the patient's family been updated on the situation and apprised of the probable negative outcome of continued resuscitation?

Summary

Asystole should be considered to be the only **true** arrhythmia because it represents a total absence of any electrical or mechanical activity in the heart. Unfortunately, asystole is frequently associated with a poor outcome.

There are, however, potentially reversible causes of asystole; therefore, a careful and systematic assessment, in addition to treating the cardiac arrest with the appropriate interventions, will maximize the chances of a successful resuscitation.

eACLS Case 3: Automated External Defibrillation (AED)

Introduction

eACLS Case 3 focuses on the management of cardiac arrest with the automated external defibrillator (AED). Most cardiac arrest patients present with ventricular fibrillation (V-Fib) as the initial cardiac dysrhythmia. V-Fib does not produce a pulse; therefore, blood is not circulated throughout the body. Pulseless ventricular tachycardia, although less common, is just as lethal as V-Fib.

The single most important treatment for these lethal ventricular dysrhythmias is early defibrillation. When effective, defibrillation "stuns" the heart, causing momentary asystole, thus allowing a dominant cardiac pacemaker to restore organized electrical activity and a perfusing rhythm.

V-Fib is a transient rhythm and rapidly deteriorates to asystole without prompt defibrillation. The AED can provide rapid defibrillation and does not require an ALS provider to operate.

The simplistic functionality of the AED requires little on the part of the rescuer other than turning on the machine, attaching the electrodes to the patient, pushing the "analyze" button, and following the directions of the AED's voice prompt.

After a brief period of analysis, the AED determines whether the patient is in a "shockable" rhythm (e.g., V-Fib or pulseless V-Tach) and informs the rescuer that a shock is advised.

Assessment and Initial Management

A careful and systematic assessment of the patient (Skill 3-1) is required in order to recognize cardiac arrest. If the patient's cardiac arrest was witnessed by you, begin CPR and apply the AED as soon as one is available. However, if the patient's cardiac arrest was not witnessed by you, perform 5 cycles (about 2 minutes) of CPR prior to applying the AED. According to the American Heart Association, return of spontaneous circulation (ROSC) occurs more often in patients with unwitnessed cardiac arrest caused by V-Fib or pulseless V-Tach if a brief period (1½ to 3 minutes) of CPR is provided before defibrillation.

Cardiac Rhythm Analysis and Defibrillation

As soon as the AED is available, it must be attached to the patient without delay (Skill 3-2). According to the American Heart Association, for each minute that V-Fib or pulseless V-Tach persists, the patient's chance of survival is reduced by approximately 10%.

If indicated, the AED will deliver a single shock, after which you should immediately perform CPR. After two minutes of CPR, reassess the patient's pulse and reanalyze his or her cardiac rhythm. If necessary, deliver another shock, followed immediately by CPR.

Summary

A rapid patient assessment is required in order to confirm the presence of cardiac arrest and begin the appropriate treatment as soon as possible.

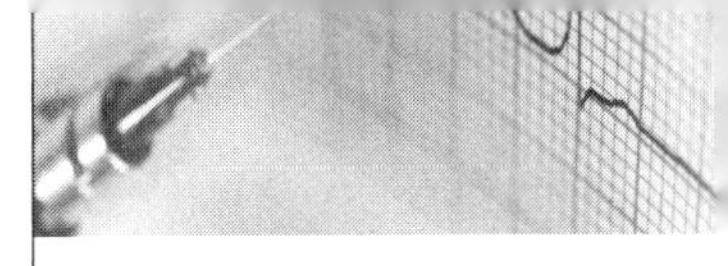

Skill 3-1: Assessment and Initial Management of Cardiac Arrest

1

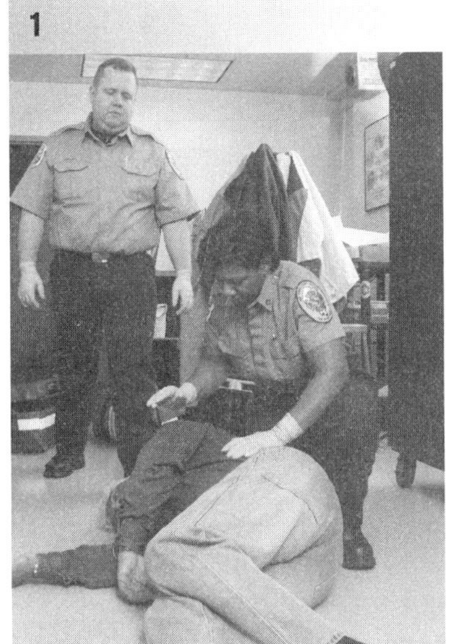

Assess for unresponsiveness.

2

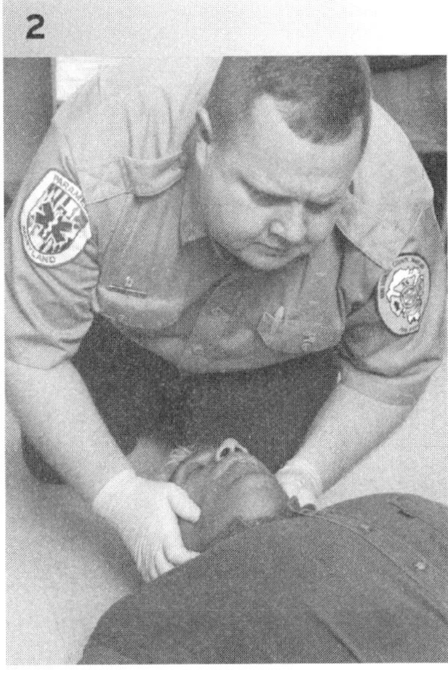

Open the airway and assess for breathing.

3

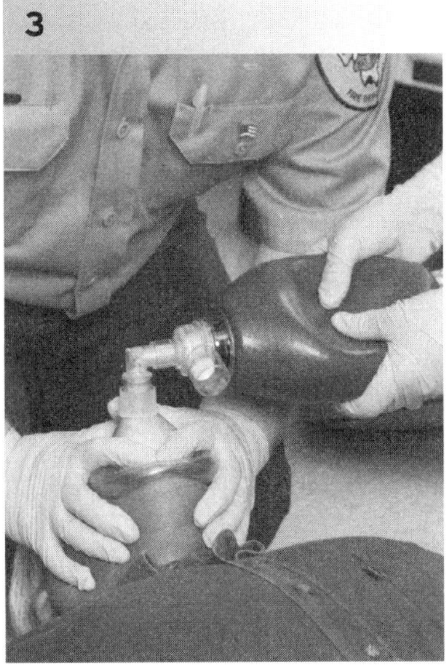

Deliver two rescue breaths.

4

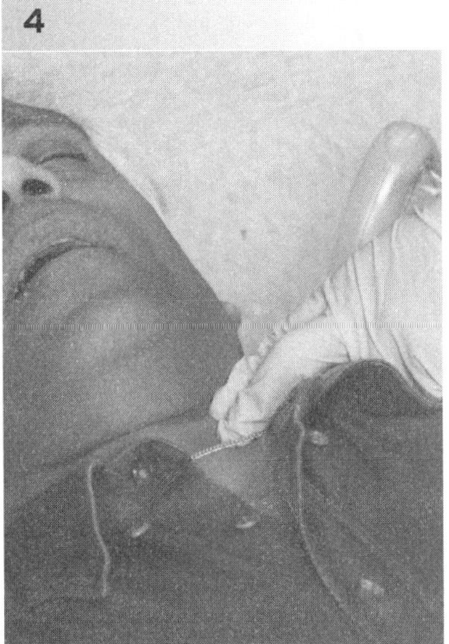

Assess for a carotid pulse.

5

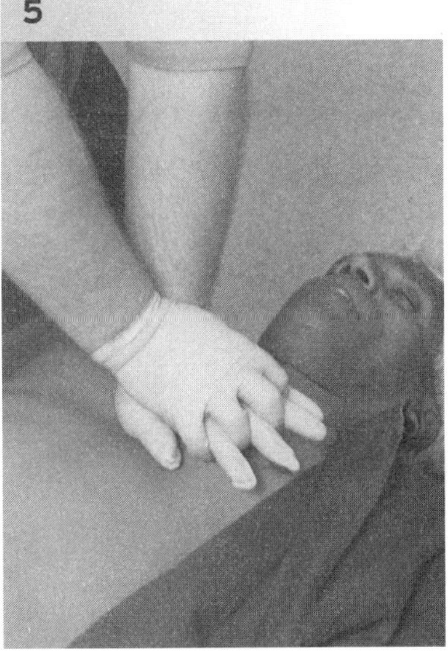

Begin CPR until the AED arrives.

If you witness the patient's cardiac arrest, begin CPR and attach the AED as soon as one is available. However, if you did not witness the patient's cardiac arrest, perform 5 cycles (about 2 minutes) of CPR before attaching the AED to the patient.

Failure to recognize and immediately treat V-Fib or pulseless V-Tach results in rapid deterioration to asystole, in which the chance of successful resuscitation is minimal.

Skill 3-2: AED Analysis and Defibrillation

1

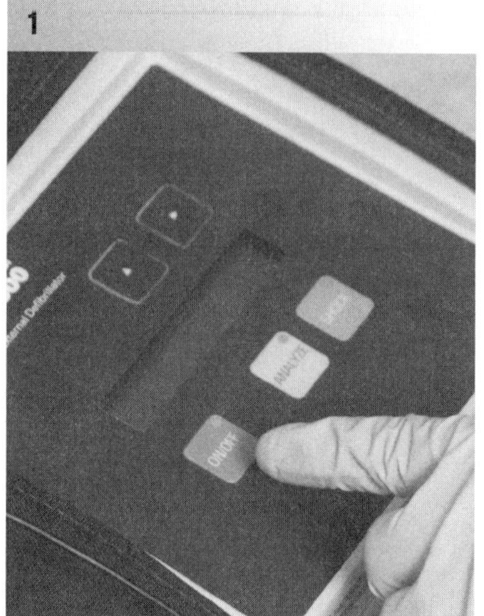

Turn the AED on.

2

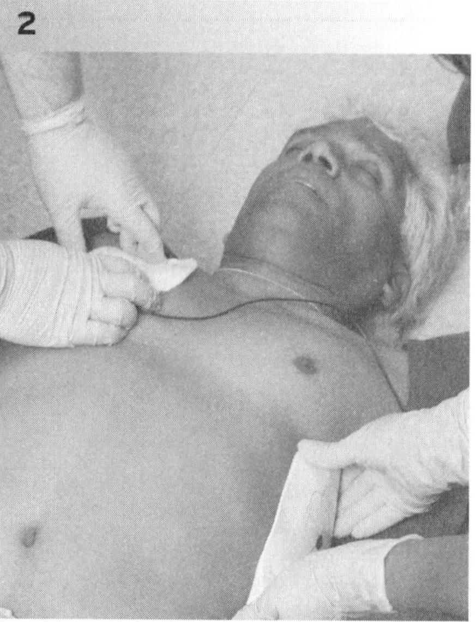

Attach the electrodes to the patient's chest.

3

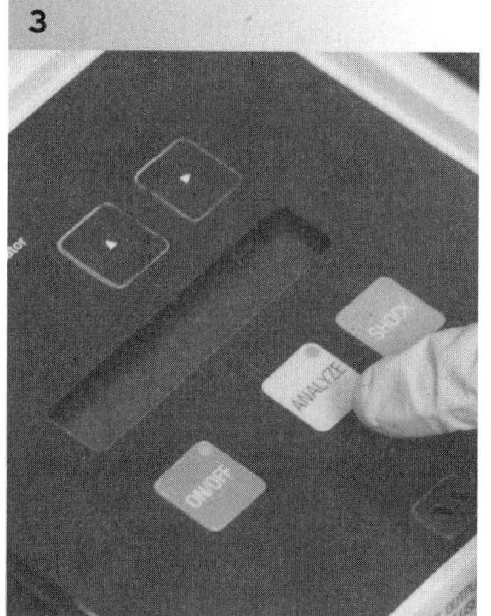

Ensure everybody is "clear" and push the "analyze" button.

4

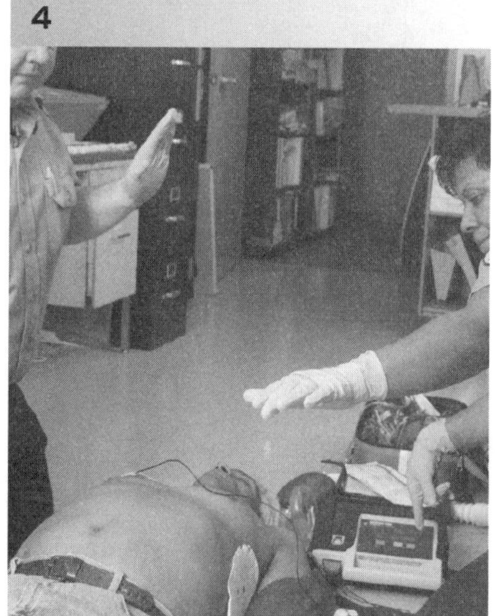

Ensure everybody is "clear" and deliver the defibrillation.

eACLS Case 4: Bradycardia

Introduction

eACLS Case 4 focuses on the assessment and management of the patient who presents with unstable bradycardia. A careful and systematic assessment must be

performed to determine whether serious signs and symptoms linked to the bradycardia are present.

Bradycardia can take on many forms, including sinus bradycardia (Figure 3-3) and varying degrees of AV heart block, such as complete (third-degree) heart block (Figure 3-4). However, the important concept to remember is that regardless of the rhythm, the rate is too slow, and if the patient is symptomatic, it must be treated.

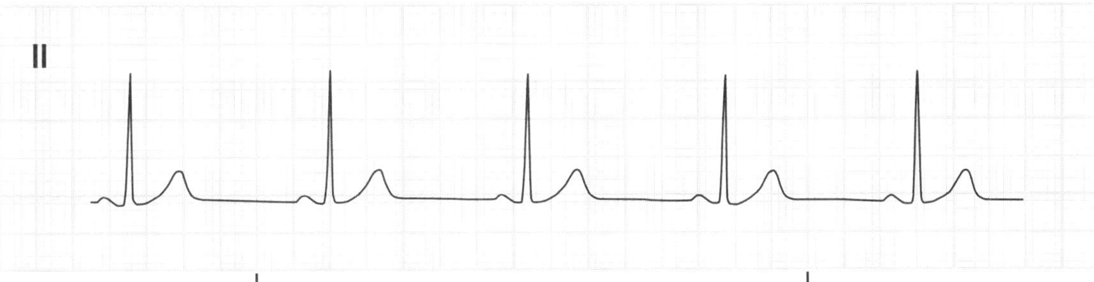

Figure 3-3: Sinus bradycardia.

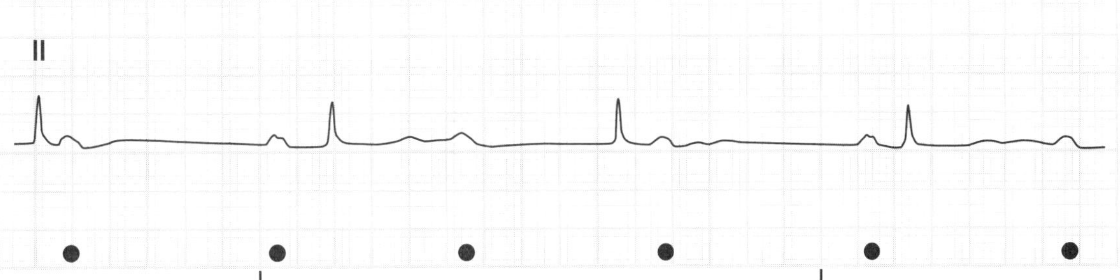

Figure 3-4: Third-degree AV block.

Absolute and Relative Bradycardia

Absolute bradycardia exists when the ventricular rate is less than 60 beats per minute, such as occurs with sinus bradycardia. Relative bradycardia exists when the patient's heart rate is faster than one would expect for his or her condition, yet the patient is unstable. For example, a patient with a heart rate of 65 beats per minute and a blood pressure of 80/50 mm Hg may be experiencing a "relative" bradycardia because the pulse rate relative to the blood pressure is too slow.

Treatment for Bradycardia

Treatment for a bradycardic rhythm depends on the presence or absence of serious signs and symptoms. The asymptomatic patient may require little more than close monitoring; however, the unstable patient requires interventions aimed at increasing the heart rate and improving perfusion (Table 3-11).

Table 3-11: Treatment for Unstable Bradycardia

- Supplemental oxygen
- Initiate IV line of normal saline
- 12-lead ECG
  - If available, a 12-lead ECG may provide more information regarding the patient's condition.
- Interventions aimed at increasing heart rate
  - Atropine, 0.5 mg via rapid IV push
    - Patients with denervated hearts, such as those who have undergone heart transplant, are not likely to respond to atropine and require immediate transcutaneous pacing (TCP).
  - TCP, if available
    - Immediate TCP should be initiated for patients with second-degree type II and third-degree AV block.
  - Epinephrine infusion at 2–10 mcg/min
  - Dopamine infusion at 2–10 mcg/kg/min
    - Consider a 500-mL normal saline bolus before giving dopamine.

Summary

The patient with bradycardia who is asymptomatic generally requires little more than monitoring. If, however, the patient presents with serious signs and symptoms linked to the bradycardia, immediate interventions aimed at increasing the heart rate and preventing cardiovascular collapse are required.

Remember that even though the patient may have a heart rate of 60–70 beats per minute, the blood pressure may be too low, which would make the patient "relatively" bradycardic and in need of the same interventions as the patient with absolute bradycardia.

eACLS Case 5: Narrow-Complex Tachycardia

Introduction

eACLS Case 5 focuses on the assessment and management of the patient who presents with a narrow-complex tachycardia. The term narrow-complex tachycardia refers to a rhythm in which the QRS complex is less than 0.12 seconds or 3 small boxes on the ECG graph paper, and a ventricular rate that is ≥ 100 beats per minute (Figure 3-5).

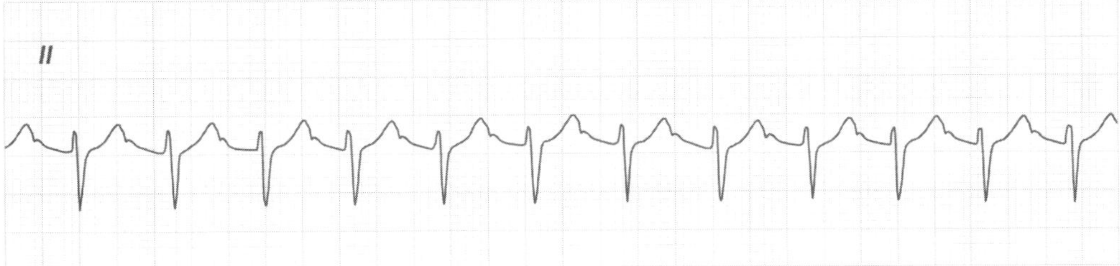

Figure 3-5: Narrow-complex tachycardia.

Supraventricular tachycardia (SVT) indicates that the origin of the cardiac rhythm is above (supra) the ventricles. SVT can include a variety of different narrow-complex tachycardias, such as atrial tachycardia, atrial fibrillation or flutter with a rapid ventricular rate (RVR), and junctional tachycardia.

Treatment for Narrow-Complex Tachycardia

A careful and systematic assessment must be performed so that the most appropriate treatment can be provided to the patient. If the patient is not experiencing serious signs and symptoms linked to the tachycardia, the initial treatment involves interventions aimed at decreasing the ventricular rate and identifying the underlying cardiac rhythm (Table 3-12).

If, however, serious signs and symptoms linked to the tachycardia exist, synchronized cardioversion (Table 3-13) must be performed without delay. Ventricular rates of less than 150 per minute typically do not require synchronized cardioversion.

Table 3-12: Treatment for Stable Narrow-Complex Tachycardia

- Supplemental oxygen
- Initiate IV line of normal saline
- Therapeutic interventions aimed at decreasing the heart rate
  - ▫ Vagal maneuvers (e.g., carotid sinus massage, valsalva)
  - ▫ Adenosine, 6 mg via rapid (over 1–3 seconds) IV push. A second dose of adenosine can be given at 12 mg, which can be repeated once (total of 30 mg).
- Pharmacologic interventions
  - ▫ Antiarrhythmics
    - Amiodarone, 150 mg IV over 10 minutes (dilute in 20–30 mL of D_5W), which may be repeated every 10 minutes as needed
    - Digoxin, 10–15 mcg/kg will provide a therapeutic effect with minimal risk of toxicity

Continued

Table 3-12: continued

- Calcium channel blockers
  - Diltiazem, 15–20 mg (0.25 mg/kg) IV push over 2 minutes, which may be repeated 15 minutes later at 20–25 mg (0.35 mg/kg) IV push over 2 minutes.
  - Verapamil, 2.5–5 mg IV over 2 minutes, which can be repeated 15–30 minutes later at 5–10 mg, to a maximum dose of 20 mg
- Beta blockers
  - Metoprolol, 5 mg via slow IV every 5 minutes, to a total of 15 mg
  - Atenolol, 5 mg via slow (over 5 minutes) IV push, which may be repeated 10 minutes later at the same dose

Table 3-13: Treatment for Unstable Narrow-Complex Tachycardia

- Provide supplemental oxygen.
- Initiate IV line of normal saline.
- Have suction and intubation equipment readily available.
- Provide sedation to the conscious patient.
  - Midazolam, 1–2.5 mg via slow IV push, or
  - Diazepam, 5–10 mg via slow IV push
- Ensure that no one is in contact with the patient.
- Push the "synch" button on the defibrillator.
- Perform synchronized cardioversion[a].
  - 100 joules initially (or biphasic equivalent[b]). If unsuccessful, repeat at 200, 300, and 360 joules, respectively.

[a] *If the patient develops V-Fib or pulseless V-Tach,* turn off the synchronizer *and defibrillate immediately.*
[b] *Biphasic cardioversion, using lower energy levels, is acceptable if it is documented to be clinically equivalent to monophasic cardioversion.*

Summary

Treatment for the patient with a narrow-complex tachycardia requires a careful and systematic assessment in order to identify serious signs and symptoms linked to the tachycardia.

All patients with narrow-complex tachycardias require supplemental oxygen, IV therapy, and cardiac monitoring. A 12-lead ECG, if available, may provide additional information regarding the narrow-complex tachycardia.

If the patient is stable, initial treatment is aimed at decreasing the heart rate with a combination of vagal maneuvers and pharmacologic interventions, which may enable you to identify the underlying cardiac rhythm and adjust further treatment accordingly.

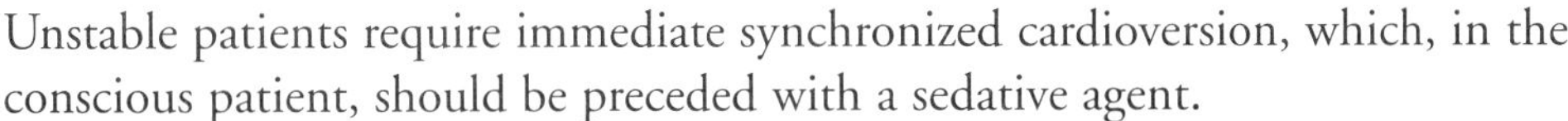

Unstable patients require immediate synchronized cardioversion, which, in the conscious patient, should be preceded with a sedative agent.

eACLS Case 6: Pulseless Electrical Activity (PEA)

Introduction

eACLS Case 6 focuses on the assessment and management of a patient who presents with pulseless electrical activity (PEA), which is characterized by a rhythm on the cardiac monitor when the patient does not have a detectable pulse. Virtually any cardiac rhythm can be seen in conjunction with PEA. The only exception to this is V-Fib and pulseless V-Tach, both of which are treated with immediate defibrillation and are not managed as PEA.

Treatment for PEA

In addition to managing the cardiac arrest itself (Table 3-14), a critical aspect in managing the patient with PEA is to focus on identifying and treating the underlying cause of the cardiac arrest. Refer to Table 3-3 (page 43) for the common causes of cardiac arrest, their clinical signs, and their respective treatments. As a general rule, rhythms that are slow indicate hypoxia, and rhythms that are fast indicate hypovolemia.

Table 3-14: Treatment for PEA

- Confirm pulselessness and apnea
  - If the arrest was witnessed, begin CPR and apply a cardiac monitor as soon as it is available.
  - If the arrest was not witnessed, perform 5 cycles (about 2 minutes) of CPR, and then apply the cardiac monitor.
- Evaluate the cardiac rhythm with defibrillator (quick-look or multipads).
- Continue CPR.
- Perform endotracheal intubation.
- Establish vascular access (IV or IO).
  - Give a 500 mL normal saline bolus, even without specific evidence of hypovolemia.
    - Hypovolemia is a very common and easily reversible cause of PEA.

Continued

Table 3-14: continued

- Administer epinephrine, 1 mg via rapid IV/IO push every 3–5 minutes.
  - Vasopressin, in a one-time dose of 40 units, may be used to replace the first or second dose of epinephrine.
  - Atropine, 1 mg via rapid IV/IO push is given every 3–5 minutes (maximum dose of 3 mg) if the pulseless cardiac rhythm is less than 60 beats per minute.
- Evaluate for and treat the underlying cause of PEA.
  - 6 Hs and 6 Ts
- Consider sodium bicarbonate, 1 mEq/kg via rapid IV/IO push.
  - Sodium bicarbonate is indicated in cases of metabolic acidosis (as evidenced by suggestive blood gas readings), tricyclic antidepressant overdose, and a prolonged (> 10 minutes) cardiac arrest interval. Sodium bicarbonate is ineffective and is potentially harmful in patients with hypercarbic acidosis.
  - Initial treatment of acidosis—regardless of the underlying cause—is to ensure adequate oxygenation and ventilation.

Summary

Pulseless electrical activity is a phenomenon that could be overlooked if you do not perform a careful assessment of your patient. It would be quite embarrassing to focus on the rhythm that the cardiac monitor is displaying, only to have someone tell you that the patient does not have a pulse!

Treatment for PEA involves treating the cardiac arrest with CPR, airway management, IV therapy, and medications. The ultimate goal is to rapidly identify and treat the underlying cause of the cardiac arrest.

eACLS Case 7: Respiratory Arrest

Introduction

eACLS Case 7 focuses on the assessment and management of the patient with respiratory arrest, including respiratory arrest caused by a foreign body airway obstruction (FBAO). You must perform a rapid assessment of the patient to identify the presence of respiratory arrest. Immediate positive-pressure ventilations must then be provided, while maintaining airway patency. Failure to recognize and immediately treat the apneic patient leads to cardiopulmonary arrest and death of the patient within minutes.

Assessment

In order to assess the patient's airway, you must first ensure that it is open and clear of secretions or obstructions. In the noninjured patient, this is accomplished by performing a head-tilt chin-lift maneuver, or, in the patient with suspected spinal injury, the jaw-thrust maneuver. It is critical that the patient's airway remain clear at all times; therefore, vomitus or other secretions in the airway require immediate oropharyngeal suctioning.

Next, assess for the presence of spontaneous breathing, as evidenced by a noted rise and fall of the chest and the sound of air exiting the nose and mouth.

Management

Initial management for the patient in respiratory arrest involves maintaining a patent airway with a combination of manual positioning of the head, and the insertion of a basic airway adjunct, such as an oropharyngeal or nasopharyngeal airway.

Positive-pressure ventilations are then provided with a bag-valve mask or a pocket mask device at a rate of 10–12 breaths per minute (1 breath every 5–6 seconds). In order to deliver high concentrations of oxygen, you must ensure that supplemental oxygen is attached to the ventilatory device you are using.

Foreign Body Airway Obstruction (FBAO)

A foreign body, such a piece of food, can obstruct the airway and prevent the patient from moving air. This phenomenon is recognized when, during your initial attempts to ventilate the patient, you meet resistance and/or do not see the chest rise. Clearly, this is a dire emergency that must be corrected immediately. Further management of the patient would clearly be futile if their airway is not patent.

If the chest does not visibly rise and/or you meet resistance during initial attempts to ventilate the patient, reposition the patient's head, and then reattempt to ventilate. If both breaths do not produce visible chest rise, perform chest compressions to attempt to dislodge the obstruction (Skill 3-3).

If chest compressions fail to dislodge the airway obstruction, visualize the vocal cords with a laryngoscope (direct laryngoscopy), and remove the obstruction with Magill forceps (Skill 3-4).

Endotracheal Intubation

In the adult patient, endotracheal intubation (Skill 3-5) is considered the "gold standard" for airway management. Patients in both respiratory and cardiac arrest usually require prolonged ventilatory support and are at an extremely high risk for regurgitation and aspiration of stomach contents; therefore, their airway should be protected with an endotracheal tube.

Skill 3-3: FBAO Removal with Abdominal Thrusts

1

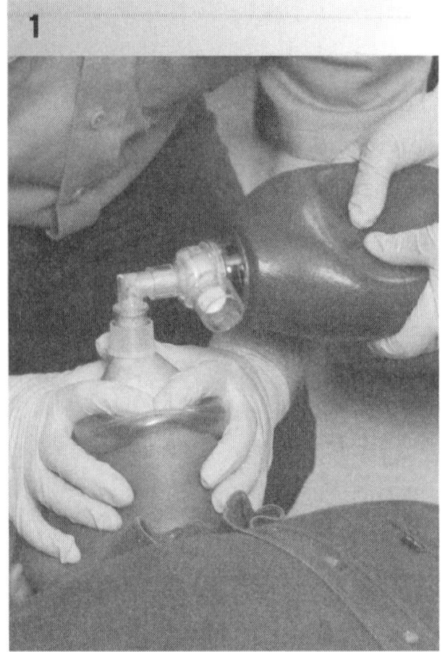

Attempt to ventilate patient.

2

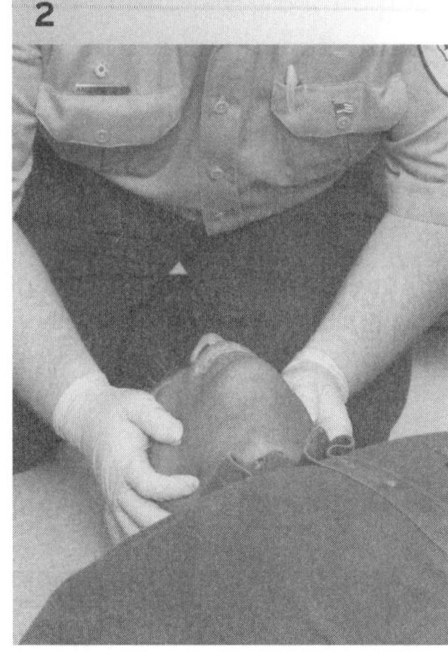

If unsuccessful, reposition the patient's head.

3

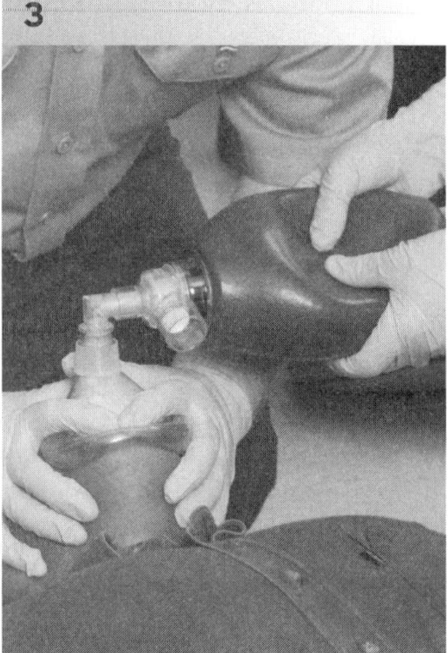

Attempt to ventilate patient again.

4

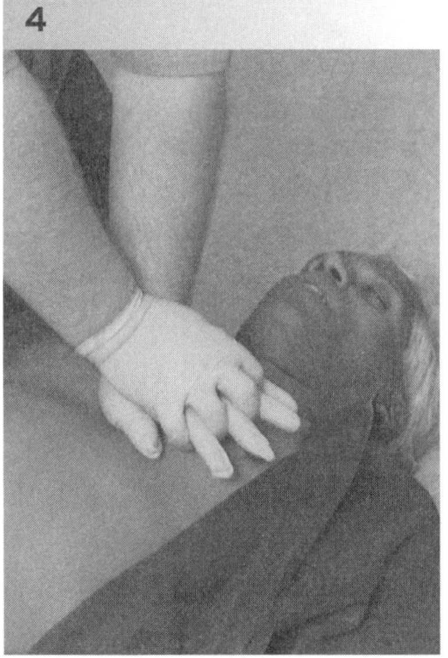

If still unsuccessful, perform 30 chest compressions.

5

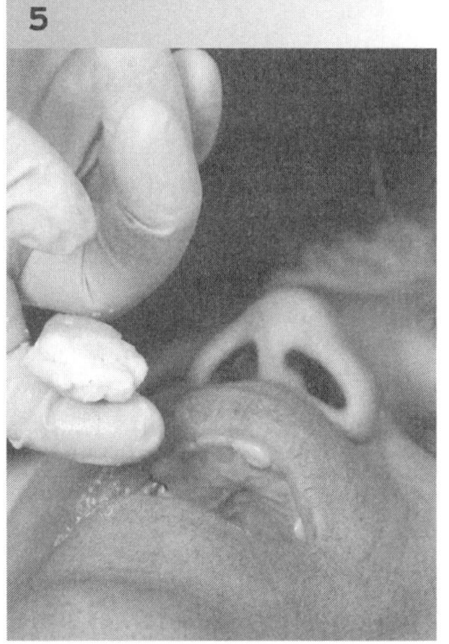

Open the airway and look in the mouth. Remove the object if it is visible.

6

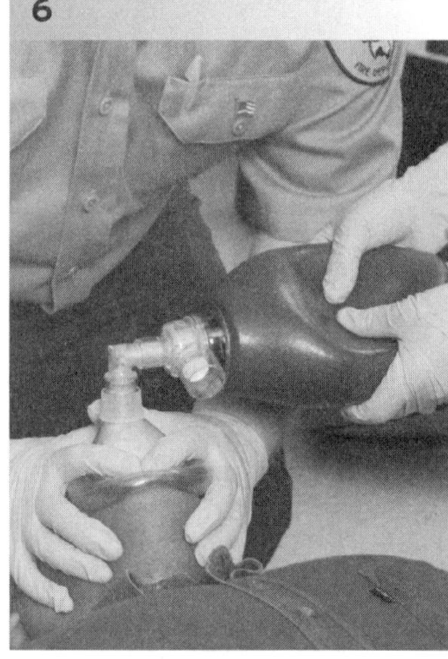

Attempt to ventilate patient.

Preoxygenation of the patient using a bag-valve mask or a pocket mask device for 2–3 minutes is a crucial step before intubation is performed. Preoxygenation provides the patient with pulmonary oxygen reserve because ventilations are interrupted during the intubation procedure.

Skill 3-4: FBAO Removal with Magill Forceps

1

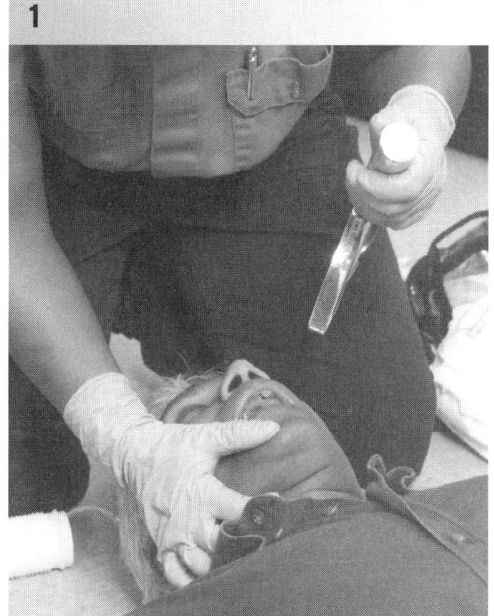

Visualize vocal cords with a laryngoscope.

2

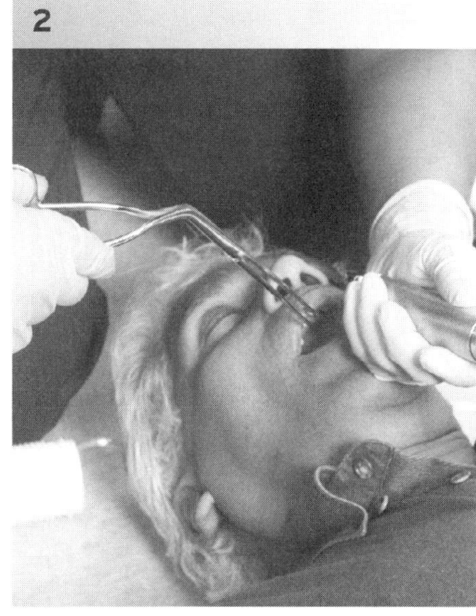

Insert Magill forceps and grasp the foreign body.

3

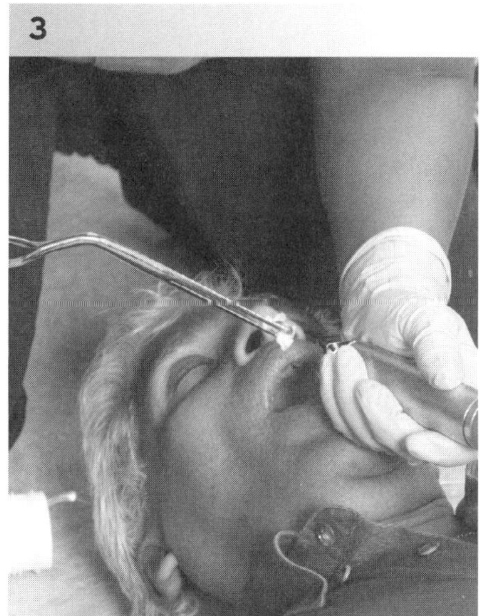

Remove foreign body.

4

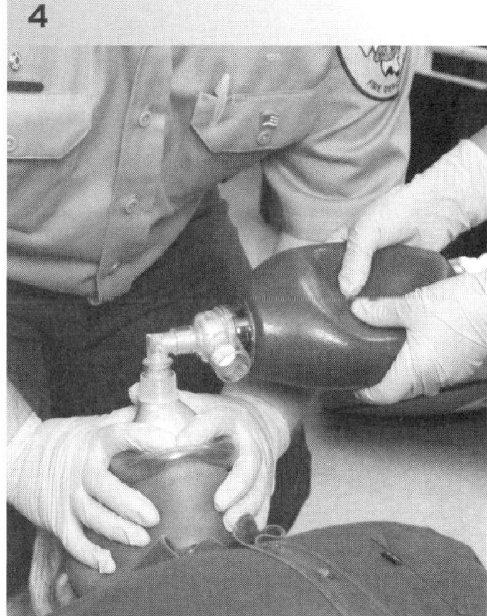

Attempt to ventilate patient.

Alternative Airway Devices

If endotracheal intubation is unsuccessful, alternative airway devices are available that enable you to secure a patent airway.

Skill 3-5: Performing Endotracheal Intubation

1

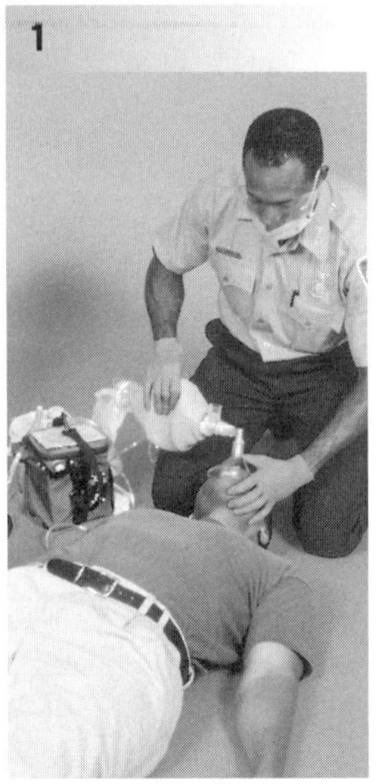

Preoxygenate the patient.

2

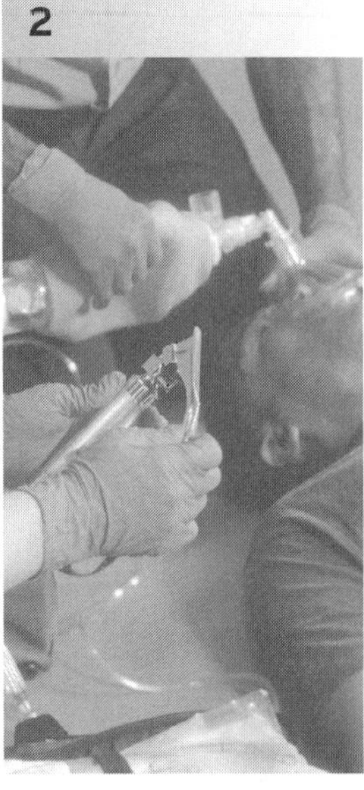

Assemble and test your equipment.

3

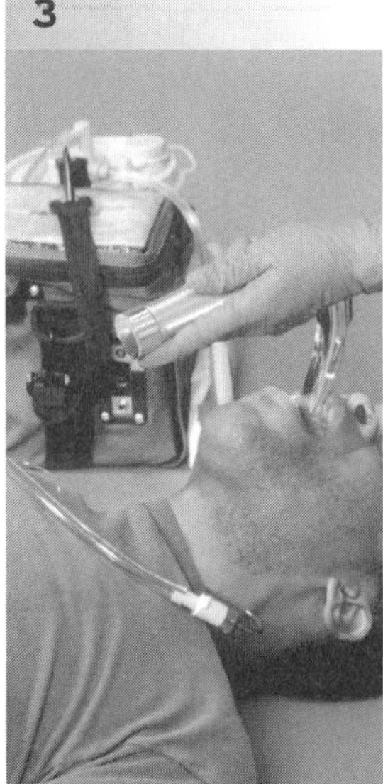

Insert the laryngoscope and visualize the vocal cords.

4

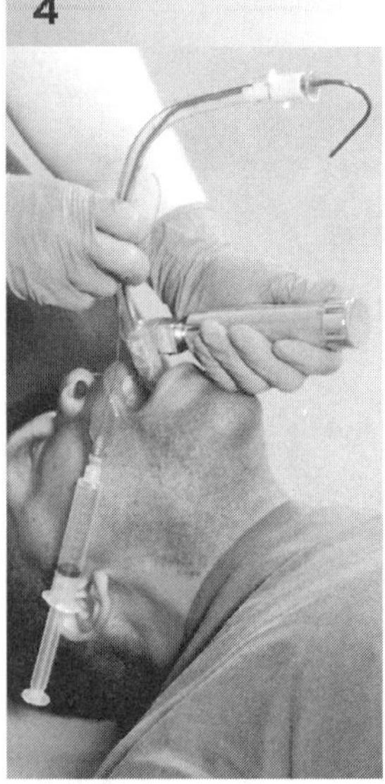

Advance the tube to the proper depth in between the vocal cords.

5

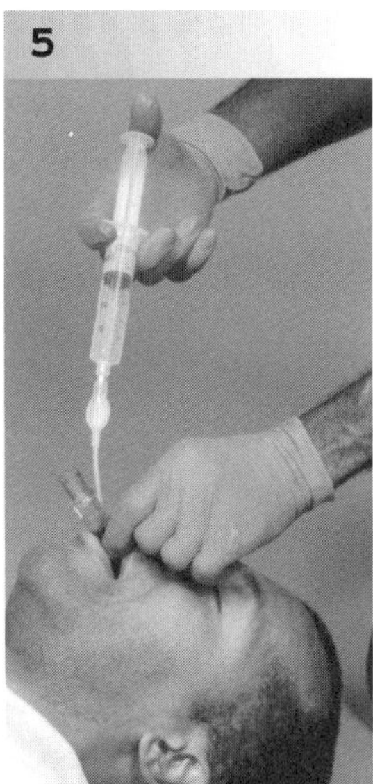

Inflate the distal cuff with 5-10 mL of air and disconnect the syringe.

6

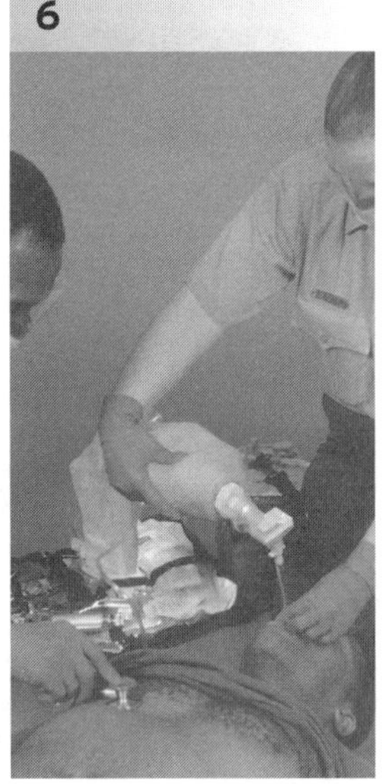

Ventilate the patient, confirm correct tube placement by auscultating over both lungs and the epigastrium, and attach an end-tidal CO_2 detector.

7

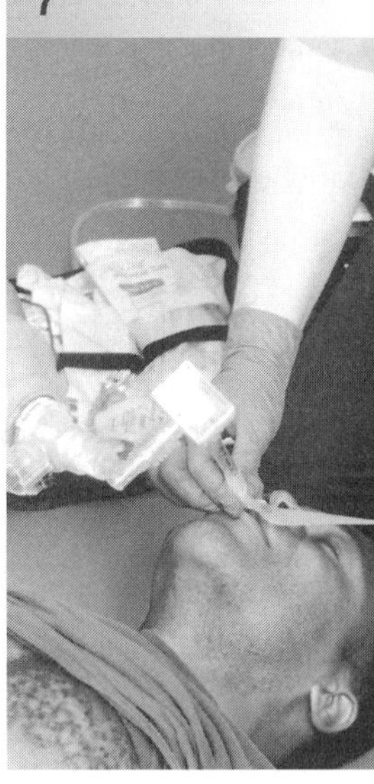

Properly secure the tube and continue to ventilate.

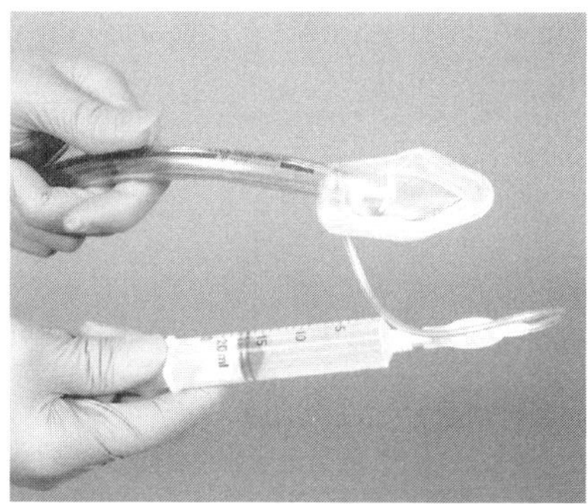

Figure 3-6: The laryngeal mask airway.

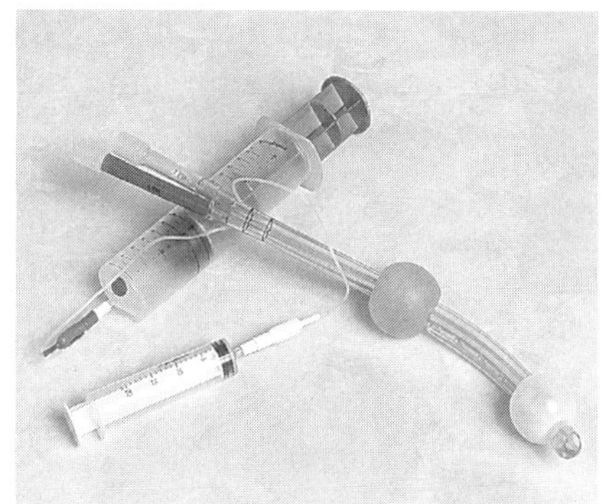

Figure 3-7: Esophageal Combitube.

The laryngeal mask airway (LMA) is a rather simplistic airway device (Figure 3-6) that is rapidly gaining popularity as an alternative to intubation. The LMA is inserted blindly into the airway while it is guided in place with the middle finger. The mask, when properly seated, covers the esophagus and facilitates air flow into the lungs.

Dual-lumen airway devices, such as the esophageal Combitube (Figure 3-7) are also acceptable alternatives to intubation. Dual-lumen devices are blindly advanced into the airway and come to rest in the esophagus in most cases. Verification of placement is accomplished by ventilating into the tube that produces clear and equal breath sounds and no epigastric sounds.

Summary

Before assessing the patient's airway, you must first ensure that it is open and clear of obstructions. After confirming the absence of breathing, provide two ventilations with a bag-valve mask or a pocket mask device.

If initial ventilations are unsuccessful, a foreign body airway obstruction is likely, and immediate corrective action must be taken to relieve the obstruction. This involves chest compressions initially, and, if necessary, removal of the obstruction with Magill forceps under direct laryngoscopy.

Once the airway is patent, continue positive-pressure ventilations at a rate of 10–12 breaths per minute (1 breath every 5–6 seconds). To definitively secure the airway, endotracheal intubation should be performed.

eACLS Case 8: Stroke

Introduction

eACLS Case 8 focuses on the assessment and management of the patient with an acute ischemic stroke. An ischemic stroke is the result of a blocked cerebral artery. Common causes include the formation of a local thrombus (Figure 3-8) or a thrombus that breaks free (embolus) and travels to the brain from another part of

the body (Figure 3-9). Less common causes of acute ischemic stroke include cerebral arterial vasospasm and generalized hypoperfusion (shock).

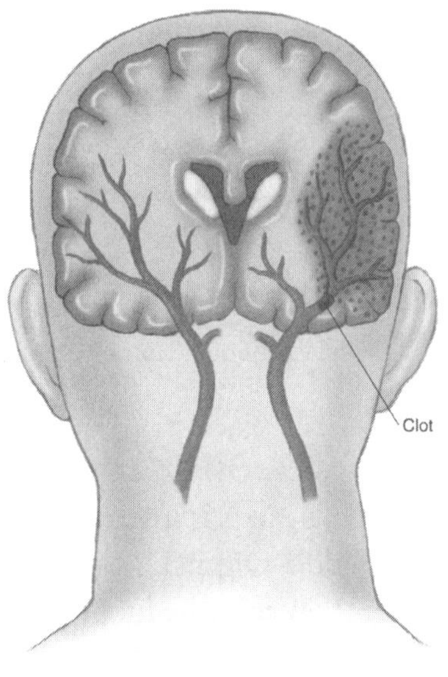

Figure 3-8: Thrombotic stroke.

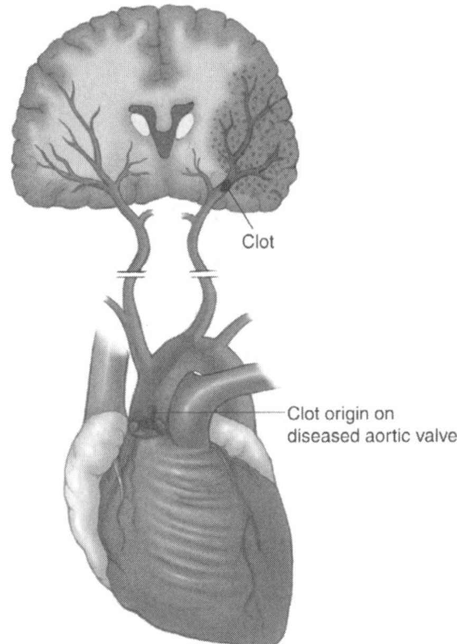

Figure 3-9: Embolic stroke.

All areas distal to the blocked artery are deprived of oxygen, resulting in varying degrees of neurologic impairment ranging from limited mobility to total debilitation.

Stroke Survival and Recovery

When caring for a stroke patient, the goal is to be able to begin therapy no more than 60 minutes from arrival at the hospital door **and** within 3 hours of the onset of the symptoms. This requires that both prehospital and hospital providers avoid any delays.

The 7 "Ds" of stroke survival and recovery (Table 3-15) represent pivotal points during the assessment and care for the stroke patient in which the highest potential for delay exists.

Table 3-15: The 7 "Ds" of Stroke Survival and Recovery

- **D**etection of stroke signs and symptoms
- **D**ispatch of EMS in a prompt manner
- **D**elivery of prehospital care by paramedics
- **D**oor-to-treatment time no longer than 60 minutes
- **D**ata collected by the physician after an exam of the patient
- **D**ecision to initiate specific stroke treatment (e.g., fibrinolytics)
- **D**rug administration as soon as the decision has been made

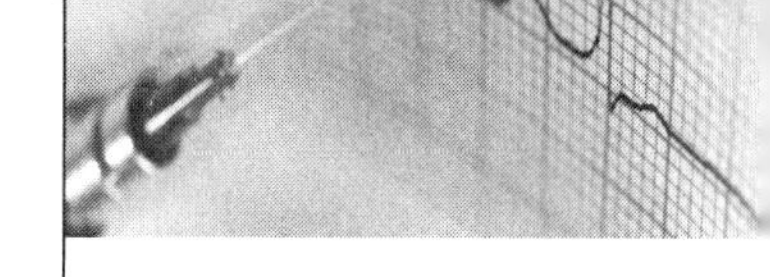

Assessment

After assessment and appropriate management of airway, breathing, and circulation, a rapid assessment of the patient and a brief, targeted history help you identify the patient's potential for having a stroke, enabling prompt treatment. The warning signs of an acute ischemic stroke include:

- Confusion
- Slurred speech (dysarthria)
- Unilateral facial droop
- Unilateral weakness or paralysis

It is particularly important to determine when the symptoms began. If the patient meets the inclusion criteria, fibrinolytic therapy can be initiated; however, this must be accomplished within 3 hours of the onset of symptoms.

Cincinnati Prehospital Stroke Scale

The Cincinnati Prehospital Stroke Scale (Table 3-16), which is used by prehospital providers, is composed of three tests to help assess whether a patient may be having a stroke. An abnormal finding in any 1 of these 3 tests indicates a high probability of a stroke.

Table 3-16: Cincinnati Prehospital Stroke Scale

- Facial droop
  - Normal: both sides of the face move equally
  - Abnormal: one side of the face does not move
- Arm drift (instruct patient to close eyes)
  - Normal: both arms move equally
  - Abnormal: one arm drifts compared with the other
- Speech
  - Normal: patient uses correct words with no slurring
  - Abnormal: patient slurs words, uses inappropriate words, or is mute

Treatment

Treatment for the stroke patient is mainly supportive and focuses on protecting the airway and delivering supplemental oxygen, monitoring the ECG, providing IV therapy, and promptly transporting or transferring the patient to a facility that specializes in stroke care, where fibrinolytic therapy can be initiated (Table 3-17).

Table 3-17: Treatment for the Stroke Patient

- Provide supplemental oxygen.
- Initiate an IV line of normal saline.
    - Avoid the use of D_5W.
- Conduct ECG monitoring.
    - Certain cardiac dysrhythmias (e.g., atrial fibrillation) can cause a stroke.
    - Monitor and treat the patient for cardiac dysrhythmias.
- Transport/transfer patient for definitive care.
    - A facility that specializes in stroke management can perform a CT scan of the head and initiate fibrinolytic therapy.

Fibrinolytic Therapy for Acute Ischemic Stroke

If the onset of symptoms of acute ischemic stroke is within 3 hours and the patient meets the inclusion criteria (Table 3-18), they may be eligible for fibrinolytic therapy. At the present time, alteplase (Activase) is the only fibrinolytic agent approved by the United States Food and Drug Administration (FDA) to treat an acute ischemic stroke. If this drug is given promptly, neurologic deficit resulting from the stroke can be minimized. Refer to Table 3-9 (page 51) for fibrinolytic exclusion criteria.

Table 3-18: Fibrinolytic Inclusion Criteria for Acute Ischemic Stroke

- Sudden onset of the following:
    - Focal neurologic deficits
        - Abnormal Cincinnati Prehospital Stroke Scale
    - Alterations in level of consciousness
- Intracranial hemorrhage ruled out with head CT
- Symptoms not rapidly improving spontaneously

Summary

An acute ischemic stroke can be a catastrophic event that can leave the patient with permanent disabilities, ranging from mild neurologic deficits to complete incapacitation. All patients with a possible acute ischemic stroke require supplemental oxygen, IV therapy, and cardiac monitoring. After a careful and systematic assessment of the patient, the clinician must act quickly, identify the patient as a candidate for fibrinolytic therapy, and transport or transfer the patient for this critical intervention.

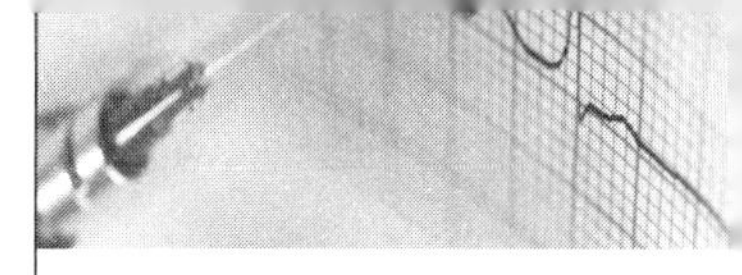

When caring for a stroke patient, the goal is to be able to begin therapy no more than 60 minutes from arrival at the hospital door **and** within 3 hours of the onset of the symptoms.

eACLS Case 9: Ventricular Fibrillation

Introduction

eACLS Case 9 focuses on the assessment and advanced management (electrical and pharmacologic) of the patient with ventricular fibrillation (V-Fib) and pulseless ventricular tachycardia (V-Tach). Basic management of these dysrhythmias was reviewed in eACLS Case 3: Automated External Defibrillation.

It is important to reiterate that for every minute V-Fib or pulseless V-Tach persists, the patient's chance of survival is reduced by 10%. The single most important treatment for V-Fib (Figure 3-10) or pulseless V-Tach (Figure 3-11) is immediate defibrillation (monophasic or biphasic equivalent).

Treatment for V-Fib and Pulseless V-Tach

The treatment algorithm for V-Fib and pulseless V-Tach (Table 3-19) assumes that the patient's condition remains unchanged. The clinician must be prepared to quickly change to the appropriate treatment algorithm on the basis of the patient's clinical response to therapy.

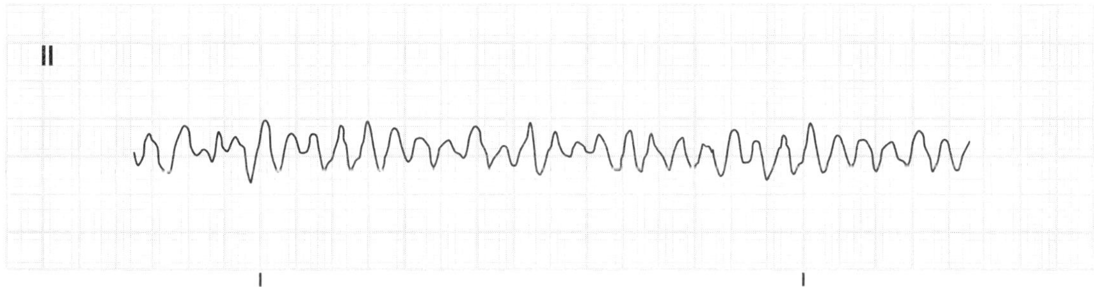

Figure 3-10: Ventricular fibrillation.

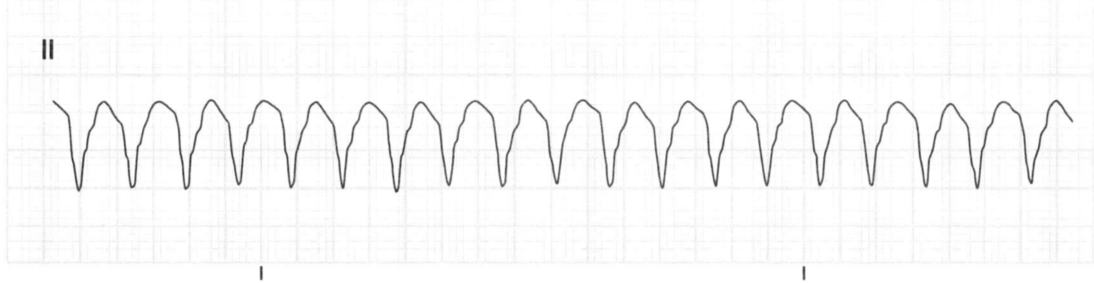

Figure 3-11: Ventricular tachycardia.

Table 3-19: Treatment for V-Fib and Pulseless V-Tach

- Confirm pulselessness and apnea.
  - If the arrest was witnessed, begin CPR and apply a cardiac monitor as soon as it is available.
  - If the arrest was not witnessed, perform 5 cycles (about 2 minutes) of CPR, and then apply the cardiac monitor.
- Evaluate the cardiac rhythm with defibrillator (quick-look or multipads).
  - Ensure that **nobody** is touching the patient.
  - Deliver one monophasic shock with 360 J (or biphasic equivalent[c]).
  - *Immediately* resume CPR.
- Perform endotracheal intubation and establish vascular access (IV or IO).
- Administer epinephrine,[d] 1 mg via rapid IV/IO push.
  - Vasopressin, in a *one-time dose* of 40 units, may be used to replace the first or second dose of epinephrine.
- Administer **one** of the following antiarrhythmic medications:
  - Amiodarone, 300 mg via rapid IV/IO push
    - Dilute in 20–30 mL of D_5W
    - May repeat dose at 150 mg diluted in 20–30 mL of D_5W 3–5 minutes later
  - Lidocaine, 1–1.5 mg/kg via rapid IV/IO push
    - May repeat dose at 0.5–0.75 mg/kg 5–10 minutes later
    - Maximum dose of 3 mg/kg

[c] *Biphasic defibrillation, using lower energy levels, is acceptable if it is documented to be clinically equivalent to monophasic defibrillation.*

[d] *Remember to circulate all drugs with effective CPR for 2 minutes, followed by defibrillation if V-Fib or pulseless V-Tach persists. Following defibrillation, immediately resume CPR and reassess the patient in 2 minutes.*

Summary

V-Fib and pulseless V-Tach are lethal dysrhythmias that do not produce a pulse or cardiac output. V-Fib is the most common initial dysrhythmia in cardiac arrest, and if it is not promptly treated, it will quickly deteriorate to asystole.

Successful management requires a rapid assessment to confirm cardiac arrest. If the patient's cardiac arrest was witnessed, begin CPR and apply a cardiac monitor as soon as one is available. If the patient's cardiac arrest was unwitnessed, perform 5

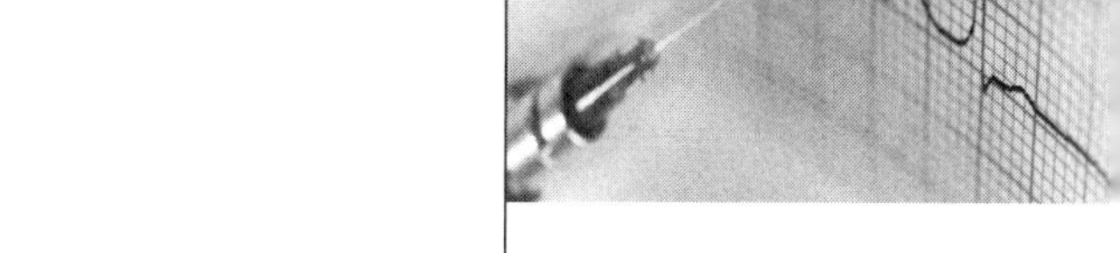

cycles (about 2 minutes) of CPR, and then apply the cardiac monitor. If V-Fib or pulseless V-Tach is present, ensure that nobody is touching the patient and defibrillate immediately.

Further management includes performing endotracheal intubation, establishing vascular access (IV or IO), and administering the appropriate pharmacologic agents.

The patient with V-Fib or pulseless V-Tach should be defibrillated one time with 360 J monophasic (or biphasic equivalent), followed immediately with CPR. After 2 minutes of CPR, reassess the patient's pulse and cardiac rhythm and defibrillate again if needed.

eACLS Case 10: Wide-Complex Tachycardia

Introduction

eACLS Case 10 focuses on the assessment and management of the patient with a wide-complex tachycardia. A wide-complex tachycardia refers to a rhythm in which the QRS complexes are greater than 0.12 seconds in width and the ventricular rate is greater than 100 beats per minute.

According to the AHA, approximately 90% of wide-complex tachycardias are ventricular tachycardia, indicating that the rhythm originated from an ectopic pacemaker in the ventricles. *Any* wide-complex tachycardia should be assumed to be ventricular tachycardia until proven otherwise.

Monomorphic ventricular tachycardia (Figure 3-12) has QRS complexes that are all of the same shape and direction. Polymorphic ventricular tachycardia (Figure 3-13), a variant of which is Torsades de Pointes, has QRS complexes that are of varying shapes and direction and resembles a combination of V-Tach and V-Fib.

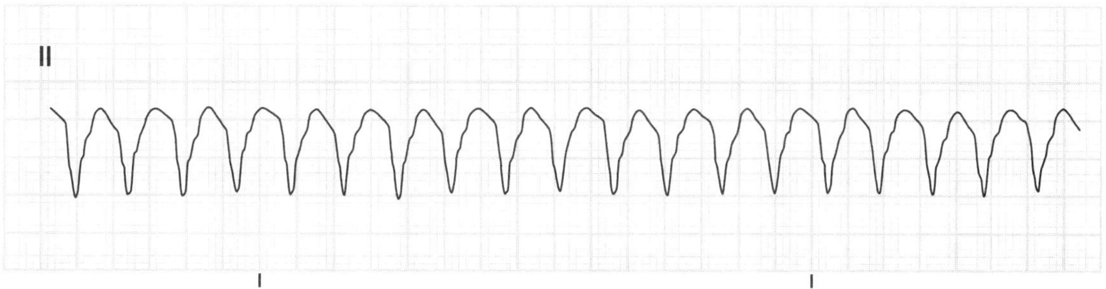

Figure 3-12: Monomorphic V-Tach.

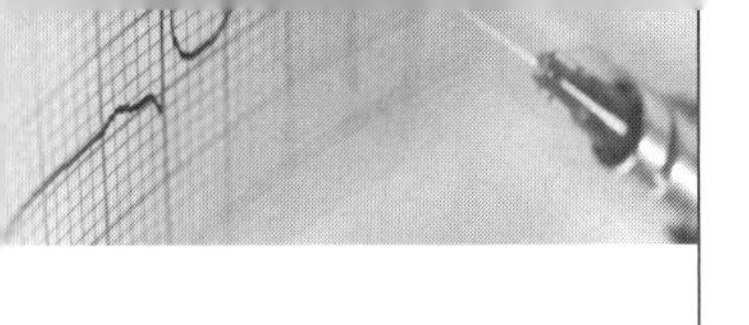

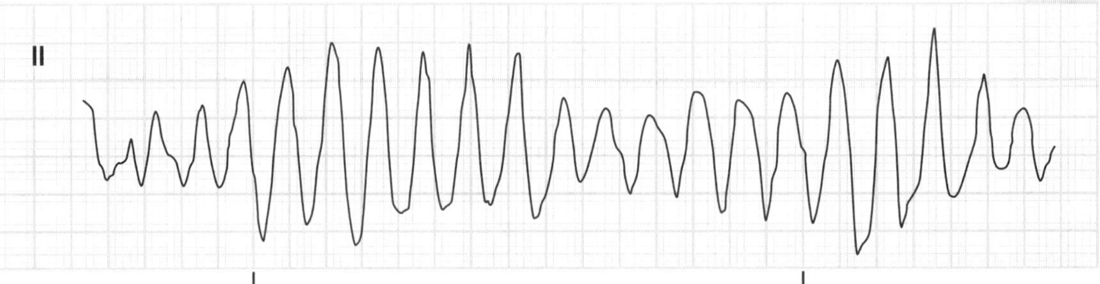

Figure 3-13: Polymorphic V-Tach.

Treatment for Wide-Complex Tachycardias

Wide-complex tachycardias (e.g., V-Tach) have a propensity for deteriorating to ventricular fibrillation and cardiac arrest. It is therefore of great importance that a careful and systematic assessment of the patient is performed in order to identify serious signs and symptoms linked to the wide-complex tachycardia, and the most appropriate treatment algorithm is selected.

If the patient is not experiencing serious signs and symptoms linked to the tachycardia, the initial treatment involves pharmacologic interventions, which are aimed at decreasing ventricular irritability, thus terminating the tachycardia (Table 3-20). *Even in the absence of serious signs and symptoms, you may elect to perform immediate synchronized cardioversion.*

If serious signs and symptoms linked to the tachycardia exist, synchronized cardioversion (Table 3-21) must be performed without delay. Because of the high risk of deterioration to V-Fib, you must be prepared to perform defibrillation if the patient becomes pulseless.

Table 3-20: Treatment for Stable Wide-Complex Tachycardias

- Provide supplemental oxygen
- IV line of normal saline
- Pharmacological interventions
    - ▫ Monomorphic V-Tach
        - Amiodarone, 150 mg IV push over 10 minutes (diluted in 20–30 mL of D_5W), which may be repeated every 10 minutes as needed
        - Lidocaine, 1–1.5 mg/kg via IV push, repeated every 5–10 minutes at 0.5–0.75 mg/kg to a maximum dose of 3 mg/kg
        - Procainamide, 20 mg/min via IV infusion until **one** of the following occurs:
            - Arrhythmia suppression.
            - Hypotension develops.

Continued

Table 3-20: continued

- QRS complex widens by > 50% of its pretreatment width
- Maximum dose of 17 mg/kg has been given

▫ Polymorphic V-Tach with *normal* QT interval

- Treat ischemia and correct electrolytes.
- Give any **one** of the following medications:
  - Amiodarone, 150 mg IV push over 10 minutes
  - Lidocaine, 1–1.5 mg/kg IV push

▫ Polymorphic V-Tach with *prolonged* QT interval

- Correct electrolyte abnormalities (e.g., hypomagnesemia, hyperkalemia).
- Magnesium sulfate, 1–2 g IV push over 5–60 minutes (dilute in 10 mL of D_5W)
- Overdrive pacing

• Electrical interventions

If V-Tach is not controlled pharmacologically, proceed with synchronized cardioversion (Table 3-21).

Table 3-21: Treatment for Unstable Wide-Complex Tachycardia

- Provide supplemental oxygen.
- Initiate IV line of normal saline.
- Have suction and intubation equipment readily available.
- Provide sedation to the conscious patient.
  - ▫ Midazolam, 1–2.5 mg via slow IV push, or
  - ▫ Diazepam, 5–10 mg via slow IV push
- Ensure that nobody is touching the patient.
- Push the "synch" button on the defibrillator.
- Perform synchronized cardioversion[e].
  - ▫ 100 J monophasic initially (or biphasic equivalent[f]). If unsuccessful, repeat at 200, 300, and 360 joules, respectively.
    - For unstable polymorphic V-Tach with a pulse, defibrillate with 360 J monophasic (or biphasic equivalent).
      - Be prepared to begin CPR if patient becomes pulseless.

[e] *If the patient develops V-Fib or pulseless V-Tach,* turn off the synchronizer *and defibrillate immediately.*

[f] *Biphasic cardioversion, using lower energy levels, is acceptable if it is documented to be clinically equivalent to monophasic cardioversion.*

Antiarrhythmic Maintenance Infusions

If a wide-complex tachycardia is pharmacologically terminated, begin a maintenance infusion of the antiarrhythmic agent that aided in the conversion (e.g., lidocaine, amiodarone, procainamide).

If synchronized cardioversion was used to terminate the wide-complex tachycardia and an antiarrhythmic agent was not administered, give a bolus of an antiarrhythmic and begin a maintenance infusion.

It is important to maintain a therapeutic blood level of the appropriate antiarrhythmic agent because this will prevent the recurrence of the wide-complex tachycardia. Refer to Chapter 2 for the appropriate antiarrhythmic maintenance infusion doses.

Summary

When a patient presents with a wide-complex tachycardia, you should assume that it is ventricular tachycardia until proven otherwise. Continuous monitoring of the patient is essential because wide-complex tachycardias can rapidly deteriorate to V-Fib.

All patients with wide-complex tachycardias require supplemental oxygen, IV therapy, and cardiac monitoring. A 12-lead ECG, if available, may provide additional information regarding the wide-complex tachycardia.

Treatment for the patient is based on whether or not they are stable (pharmacologic) or unstable (cardioversion); therefore, the clinician must perform a careful and systematic assessment of the patient to identify serious signs and symptoms linked to the wide-complex tachycardia.

Chapter 4

eACLS Practice Cases

Introduction

This chapter of the eACLS study guide presents 10 practice cases that are designed to prepare you for the interactive case simulations in the eACLS program. The practice cases are arranged randomly, thus requiring you to identify the patient's cardiac rhythm, to determine whether the patient is stable or unstable, and to administer the appropriate treatment.

For each practice case, pertinent patient assessment information, including chief complaint, ECG rhythms, vital signs, and physical exam findings, is provided. This assessment information will enable you to answer the treatment-related questions that are asked throughout the case.

Questions with a higher degree of difficulty will be labeled **"Beyond eACLS Basics"** and are intended to assess a more in-depth knowledge of the patient's condition. A summary, which contains the answers and rationales to the case questions, follows each respective practice case.

eACLS Practice Case 1

A conscious and alert 50-year-old man complains of a sudden onset of palpitations and lightheadedness, which began approximately 30 minutes previously. Currently, the patient denies chest pain or shortness of breath. The pulse oximeter reads 98% on room air.

Question 1: What initial treatment is indicated for this patient?

The initial treatment for this patient is complete. As your assistant prepares to initiate an IV line of normal saline, you attach the ECG leads to the patient's chest and assess his cardiac rhythm (Figure 4-1).

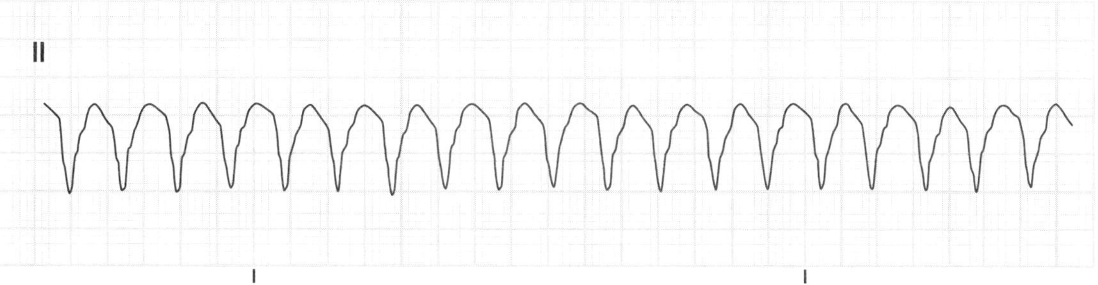

Figure 4-1: Your patient's cardiac rhythm.

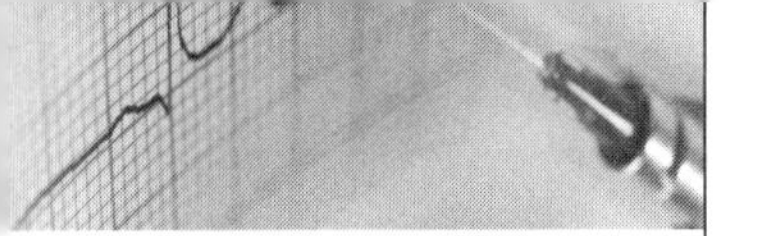

Question 2: What is your interpretation of this cardiac rhythm?

The patient's blood pressure is 138/78 mm Hg. The pulse is 182 bpm and is strong, and respirations are 20 breaths per minute and unlabored. Further assessment reveals that the patient's breath sounds are clear and equal bilaterally, and his jugular veins are normal. Your assistant reports that the IV line is patent and running at a "keep vein open" (KVO) rate.

Question 3: What treatment is indicated for this patient's condition?

You have just performed the appropriate intervention for the patient's condition when you noted a marked decrease in his level of consciousness. You immediately reassess his blood pressure, which is 80/50 mm Hg. His skin is diaphoretic, and his breathing is labored. He is placed on a nonrebreathing mask at 15 L/min.

Question 4: How will you treat this patient now?

The patient's condition remains unchanged after your next intervention. After repeating this intervention, you note a change in his cardiac rhythm (Figure 4-2).

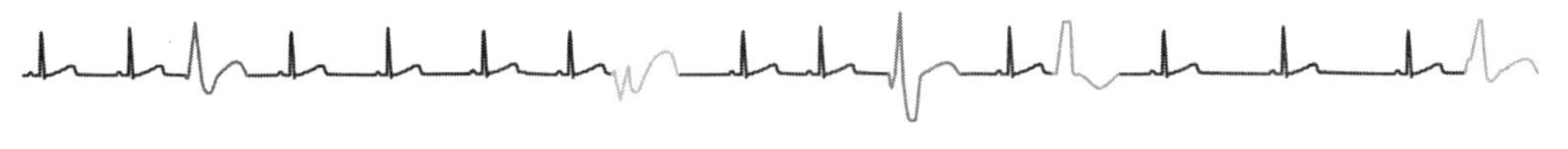

Figure 4-2: The patient's cardiac rhythm has changed.

An immediate reassessment of the patient reveals that his mental status has improved. His blood pressure is 130/70 mm Hg, and his respirations are 18 breaths per minute and unlabored. You prepare to initiate a treatment that is aimed at preventing a recurrence of his dysrhythmia.

Question 5: What will prevent a recurrence of his dysrhythmia?

The patient remains conscious and alert, and his vital signs are stable. His cardiac rhythm now reveals a normal sinus rhythm. With continuous monitoring, you transfer the patient for continued care.

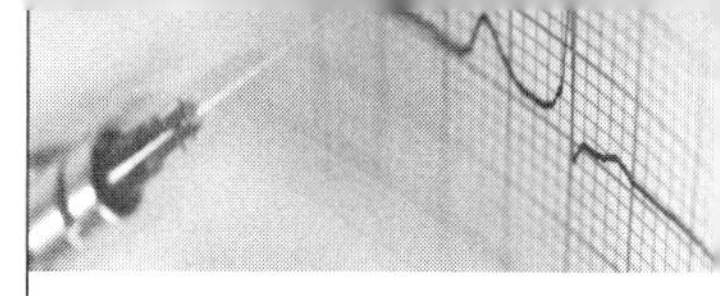

Beyond eACLS Basics: What specific treatment would be required if this patient's potassium level was severely low (less than 2 mEq/L)?

eACLS Practice Case 1 Summary

Question 1: What initial treatment is indicated for this patient?
The patient is not exhibiting signs of significant hypoxia, and his oxygen saturation is 98%. Supplemental oxygen via a nasal cannula at 4 L/min would be appropriate.

Oxygen is the first drug that is administered to patients with a cardiovascular or respiratory system emergency. Sufficient concentrations should be given to maintain oxygen saturations of greater than 90%. A nonrebreathing mask should be applied if signs of hypoxia (e.g., cyanosis, altered level of consciousness) are present.

Question 2: What is your interpretation of this cardiac rhythm?

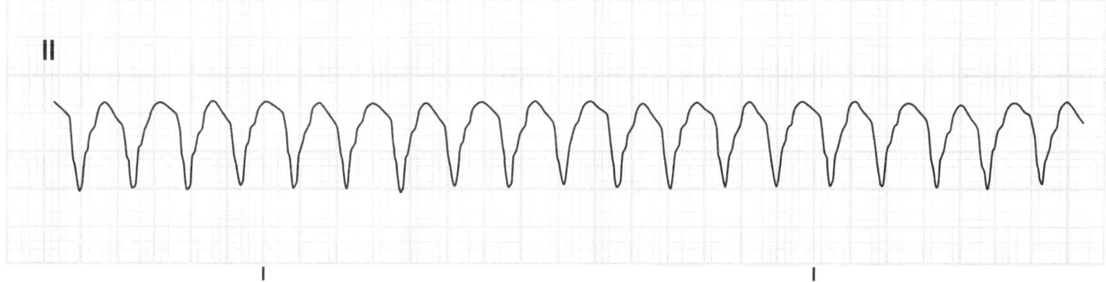

The cardiac rhythm depicted is monomorphic V-Tach. The rhythm is regular with a rate of approximately 180 beats per minute. The QRS complexes are wide and bizarre, and there are no discernable P waves. The term "monomorphic" means that all of the QRS complexes are the same size, shape, and direction.

V-Tach indicates the presence of an irritable ectopic focus in the ventricles that has become the dominant cardiac pacemaker. If not treated promptly, V-Tach could deteriorate to V-Fib and cardiac arrest.

Question 3: What treatment is indicated for this patient's condition?
This patient is not exhibiting serious signs and symptoms that are linked to his V-Tach; therefore, he is considered stable. Treatment with an antiarrhythmic agent is appropriate at this point. Any one of the following medications can be administered:

- Amiodarone: 150 mg can be given via an IV push over 10 minutes.
  - Predilute amiodarone in 20–30 mL of D_5W.
  - Repeat this same dose every 10 minutes as needed.

- Lidocaine: 1–1.5 mg/kg can be given via an IV push.
  - The repeat dose is 0.5–0.75 mg/kg every 5–10 minutes as needed.
  - Maximum dose is 3 mg/kg.
- Procainamide: 20 mg/min is given via an IV infusion.
  - Chapter 2 discusses further dosing information.

Question 4: How will you treat this patient now?
This patient's condition has clearly taken a turn for the worse. His altered mental status, hypotension, and labored respirations are serious signs and symptoms that indicate hemodynamic instability. After sedating the patient with 2.5 mg of midazolam, you must perform immediate synchronized cardioversion starting with 100 joules. If needed, repeat cardioversion at 200, 300, and 360 joules.

Question 5: What treatment will prevent recurrence of his dysrhythmia?

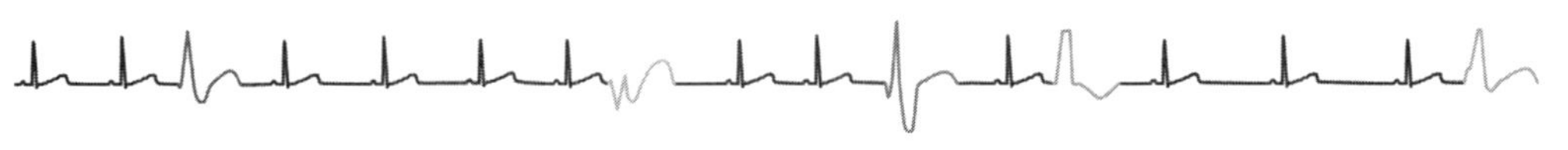

This patient is now in a sinus rhythm with multiformed premature ventricular complexes (PVCs), which indicates continued ventricular irritability and the risk of recurrent V-Tach. An antiarrhythmic maintenance infusion will help to prevent recurrent V-Tach. A bolus dose (see previously mentioned doses) must be given before beginning a maintenance infusion. Any one of the following can be used:

- Amiodarone: 1 mg/min for the first 6 hours, followed by 0.5 mg/min for the remaining 18 hours (the maximum cumulative dose is 2.2 g in 24 hours)
- Lidocaine: 1–4 mg/min titrated to the desired effect
- Procainamide: 1–4 mg/min titrated to the desired effect

Beyond eACLS Basics: What specific treatment would be required if this patient's potassium level was severely low (less than 2 mEq/L)?
Normal serum potassium levels range from 2.5–5 mEq/L. Potassium levels that are less than 2 mEq/L are often associated with QRS widening, ventricular dysrhythmias, PEA, and asystole.

Specific treatment for hypokalemia-induced V-Tach includes the administration of potassium chloride (KCl). Begin the initial infusion at 2 mEq/min over 10 minutes (20 mEq total), followed by 1 mEq/min over the next 10 minutes (10 mEq total). The infusion should be reduced carefully when the patient's condition improves.

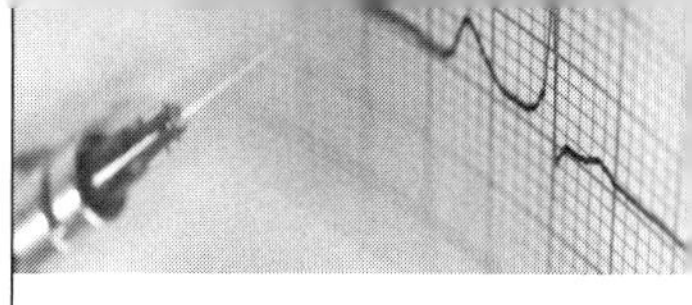

eACLS Practice Case 2

A 45-year-old female presents with shortness of breath and nausea that began 45 minutes earlier. She is conscious, although confused. You palpate her radial pulse and find that it is slow and weak. After placing her on supplemental oxygen, you assess her cardiac rhythm (Figure 4-3).

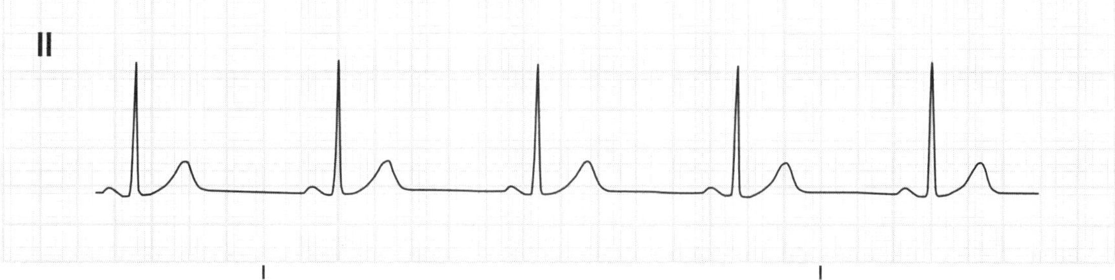

Figure 4-3: Your patient's cardiac rhythm.

Your patient has a blood pressure of 78/56 mm Hg, a pulse rate of 48 bpm weak and regular, and respirations of 24 breaths per minute and labored. Her breath sounds reveal scattered rales bilaterally. An IV line of normal saline is initiated and set at a KVO rate.

Question 1: What pharmacologic agent is indicated for this patient?

The patient's condition remains unchanged, despite having given her the maximum dose of the indicated pharmacologic agent. Your assistant urgently turns your attention to the patient's cardiac rhythm, which has changed (Figure 4-4).

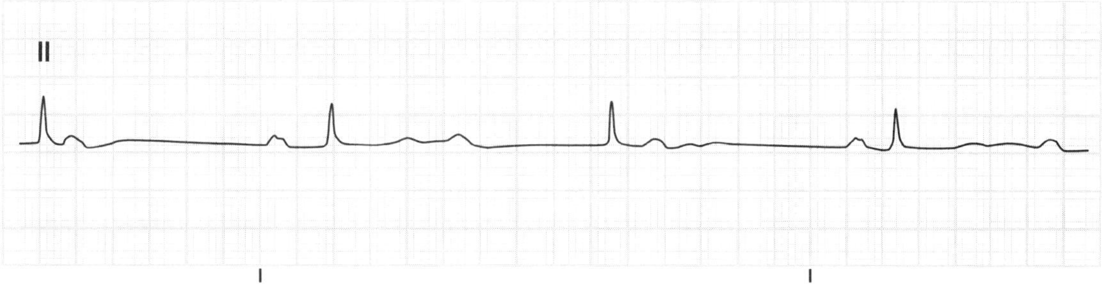

Figure 4-4: Your patient's cardiac rhythm has changed.

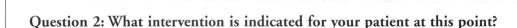

Question 2: What intervention is indicated for your patient at this point?

Your next intervention has improved the patient's cardiac rhythm (Figure 4-5). Her pulse rate corresponds with the heart rate of her cardiac rhythm.

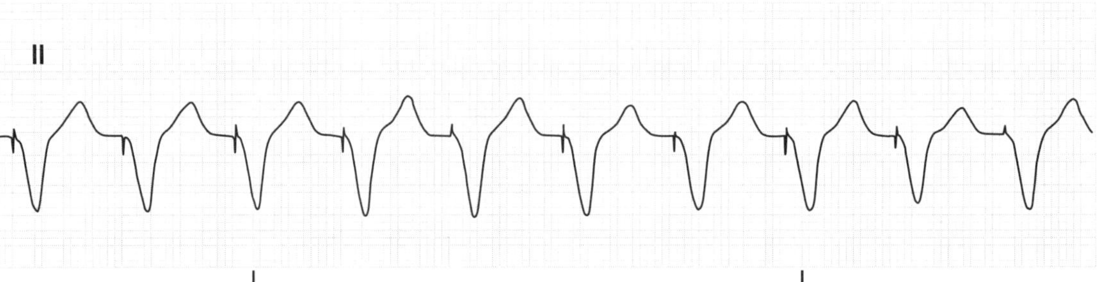

Figure 4-5: Your patient's cardiac rhythm has improved.

Although her cardiac rhythm has been corrected, the patient remains hypotensive. After a 500-mL bolus of normal saline fails to increase her blood pressure, you consider the next treatment option.

Question 3: What medication is indicated first for nonhypovolemic hypotension?

The patient's blood pressure is now 108/68 mm Hg, and her pulse rate is 84 bpm and strong. She is conscious and alert, and the pulse oximeter reads 98% on the supplemental oxygen.

Question 4: What other medication could have been used to treat this patient's hypotension?

The patient's condition continues to improve. You transfer her for more definitive care while carefully monitoring her cardiac rhythm and vital signs.

Beyond eACLS Basics: How would your treatment have differed had this been a heart transplant patient?

eACLS Practice Case 2 Summary

Question 1: What pharmacologic agent is indicated for this patient?
The patient is displaying sinus bradycardia with a rate of approximately 50 beats per minute. The rhythm is accompanied by serious signs and symptoms such as shortness of breath, hypotension, and an altered mental status, all of which her slow heart rate is causing. The first pharmacologic agent indicated for her condition is atropine sulfate 0.5 mg via a rapid IV push, which may be repeated every 3–5 minutes to a maximum vagolytic dose of 3 mg.

Question 2: What intervention is indicated for your patient at this point?

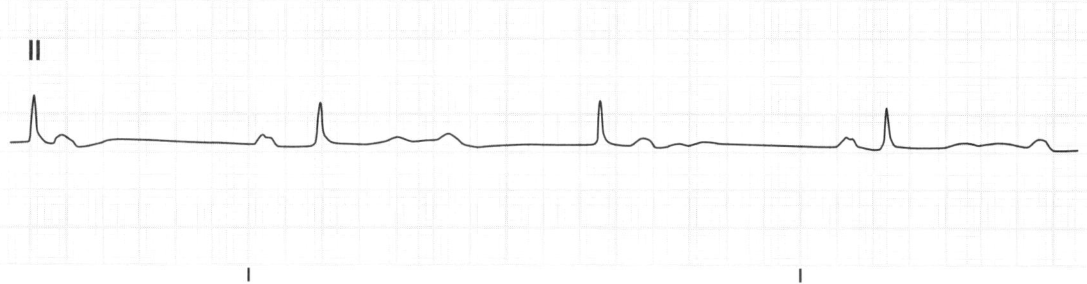

Your patient is now in a third-degree AV block, which represents total AV dissociation. The treatment of choice for this cardiac rhythm is TCP, which serves as a bridge device until a transvenous pacemaker can be inserted or a permanent pacemaker can be implanted. Drugs such as atropine are typically ineffective in treating a third-degree AV block.

Question 3: What medication is indicated first for nonhypovolemic hypotension?
Hypotension that persists despite IV fluid boluses is treated with a dopamine infusion. The dose for dopamine ranges from 2–20 mcg/kg/min. It would be most appropriate to begin the infusion at 5 mcg/kg/min and titrate up to 10 mcg/kg/min or until the desired effect is achieved. For severe hypotension, doses of greater than 10 mcg/kg/min may be needed.

Question 4: What other medication could have been used to treat this patient's hypotension?
Had dopamine been unsuccessful in raising this patient's blood pressure, an epinephrine infusion would have been the next drug of choice. The correct dose for epinephrine ranges from 2–10 mcg/min, and it is titrated to the desired effect.

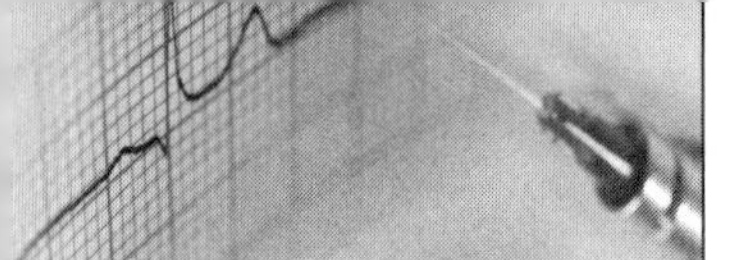

Beyond eACLS Basics: How would your treatment have differed had this been a heart transplant patient?

A transplanted heart does not have an inherent electrical conduction system; it has been denervated and is artificially paced. Atropine would not be effective, as it increases the heart rate by blocking the parasympathetic nervous system via the vagus nerve, which the denervated heart does not have. Initial treatment, therefore, would have been immediate TCP.

eACLS Practice Case 3

A 60-year-old man is found to be unconscious and cyanotic. After excluding trauma, you open his airway with a head-tilt chin-lift maneuver, assess for breathing, and determine that he is apneic. You attempt to ventilate the patient with a pocket mask device; however, the chest does not rise, and resistance is met.

Question 1: How will you initially remedy this problem?

____

____

Your initial intervention has remedied the problem, and your ventilations now produce a bilateral rise of the patient's chest. After assessing for a carotid pulse, you note that it is present. Your partner prepares additional equipment.

Question 2: How will you continue to treat this patient?

____

____

The appropriate treatment is continued. Your assistant informs you that he must perform ET intubation because the patient's cyanosis is worsening. As he is gathering the appropriate equipment, you preoxygenate the patient with 100% oxygen.

Question 3: When is ET intubation indicated in the apneic patient?

____

____

Your partner has just placed the ET tube. The distal cuff is inflated, and ventilations are continued. Auscultation reveals negative epigastric sounds and bilaterally equal breath sounds.

Question 4: What are additional methods of confirming successful intubation?

____

____

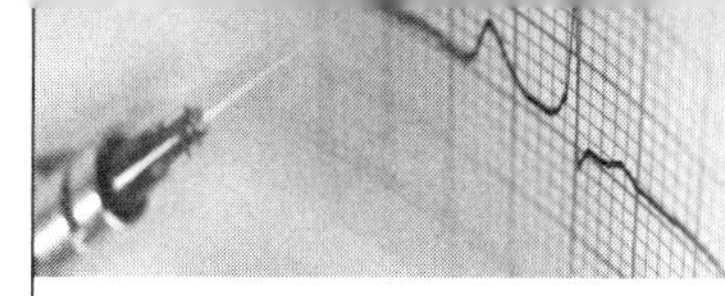

Correct ET tube placement has been confirmed with an appropriate additional method, and ventilations with 100% oxygen are continued at a rate of 10–12 breaths per minute. The patient's pulse rate, which was initially rapid, has decreased to a normal rate. His skin is now pink.

Question 5: What is the correct ventilatory duration and tidal volume for an intubated adult?

____

____

The patient is placed on a mechanical ventilator, and the rate and tidal volume are set accordingly. He is transferred for continued care, where an assessment to determine the cause of his respiratory arrest is performed.

Beyond eACLS Basics: What are the hazards of hyperventilating an apneic patient?

eACLS Practice Case 3 Summary

Question 1: How will you initially remedy this problem?
If initial ventilation attempts fail to produce a chest rise or if you meet resistance, your initial intervention is to reposition the patient's head and reattempt to ventilate. Often, the patient's head was not placed in the appropriate position initially.

Question 2: How will continue to treat this patient?
This patient is in respiratory arrest with a pulse. You must treat this patient by providing positive pressure ventilations at a rate of 10–12 breaths per minute (1 breath every 5–6 seconds) with a bag-valve mask or a pocket mask device that is attached to 100% oxygen.

Question 3: When is ET intubation indicated in the apneic patient?
Initial ventilations for an apneic patient should be provided with basic methods, such as a bag-valve mask or a pocket mask device. If, however, the rescuer is unable to ventilate with basic methods, ET intubation must be performed to secure the patient's airway. The patient in this case is remaining cyanotic despite positive pressure ventilations, which indicates ineffective bag-valve mask ventilation.

Question 4: What are additional methods of confirming successful intubation?
The end-tidal CO_2 detector, or capnographer, is a device that connects inline between the ventilatory device and the ET tube. Colorimetric paper within the end-tidal CO_2 detector should turn yellow during the exhalation phase. If the paper turns purple, the ET tube is likely in the esophagus.

The esophageal detector device is a bulb device that is squeezed, connected to the standard 15/22 mm adaptor on the ET tube, and then released. If the bulb refills

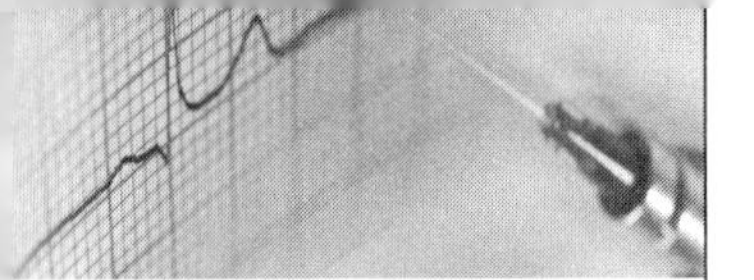

with air, the tube is likely in the trachea. If it does not refill with air, the tube is likely in the esophagus.

A chest x-ray will show the exact position of the ET tube, which should be just above the level of the carina. Although not the quickest, a chest x-ray is the most reliable method of determining correct tube placement.

Question 5: What is the correct ventilatory duration and tidal volume for an intubated adult?
When the adult patient is intubated or you are using a bag-valve-mask device, the duration of each ventilation should be 1 second, just enough to produce visible chest rise. The exact tidal volume required to achieve this varies from person to person, but is generally about 500 mL per breath in the adult.

Beyond eACLS Basics: What are the hazards of hyperventilating an apneic patient?
Hyperventilation of the apneic patient has been shown to cause several negative effects. These include increased intrathoracic pressure, which reduces cardiac output by impeding venous return to the right side of the heart, decreased cerebral perfusion pressure secondary to hyperventilation-induced cerebral vasoconstriction, and an "auto-positive-end expiratory pressure (PEEP)" effect, which is caused by inadequate exhalation and leads to air trapping in the lungs.

eACLS Practice Case 4

A 59-year-old male is found unconscious and cyanotic. Your assessment reveals that he is pulseless and apneic. Since the patient's cardiac arrest was not witnessed, you perform 2 minutes of CPR as your partner retrieves the AED. Following 2 minutes of CPR, your partner attaches the AED electrodes to the patient's chest.

Question 1: What must you do before analyzing this patient's cardiac rhythm?

____

____

The AED states "shock advised." After delivering one shock, you immediately resume CPR. Your partner quickly gathers additional equipment.

Question 2: What is your next course of action?

____

____

After 2 minutes of additional treatment, you reanalyze the patient's cardiac rhythm and receive a "check patient" message. The patient is still pulseless and apneic.

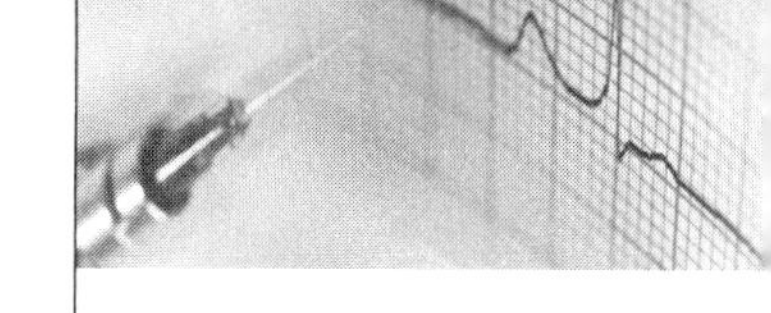

Question 3: Why would the AED give a "check patient" message?

You check the patient as directed and reanalyze his cardiac rhythm. After receiving a "shock advised" message, you ensure that both you and your partner are clear of the patient, deliver the shock, and immediately resume CPR. Following 2 minutes of CPR, you reanalyze the patient's cardiac rhythm and receive a "no shock advised" message.

Question 4: What must you do after receiving a "no shock advised" message?

A carotid pulse has been restored, but the patient remains apneic. Your partner continues providing positive-pressure ventilations at 10–12 breaths per minute as you prepare to transfer the patient for advanced life support care.

Question 5: What should you do if this patient rearrests in your presence?

After advanced life support interventions, the patient's condition continues to improve. Within 15 minutes after spontaneous circulation was restored, he has regained spontaneous breathing and is now awake.

Beyond eACLS Basics: How should you place the AED electrodes in patients with an automated implanted cardioverter/defibrillator (AICD)?

eACLS Practice Case 4 Summary

Question 1: What must you do before analyzing this patient's cardiac rhythm?
You must ensure that no one is touching the patient. The AED will not analyze the patient's cardiac rhythm if movement is detected; therefore, all contact with the patient must cease.

Question 2: What is your next course of action?
Following defibrillation, you should *immediately* resume CPR for 2 minutes. During this time, an airway adjunct should be inserted, and ventilations should be initiated with a bag-valve-mask or a pocket mask device. Be sure to attach supplemental oxygen to the ventilatory device that you are using. Following 2 minutes of CPR, you should reanalyze the patient's cardiac rhythm.

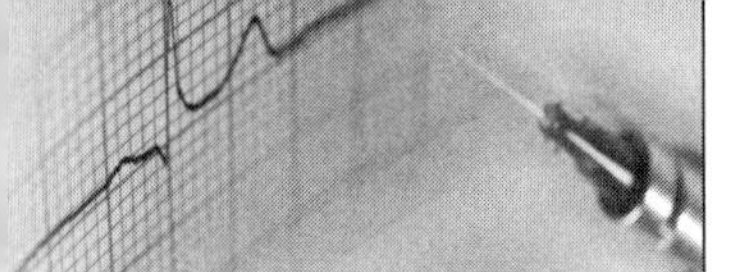

Question 3: Why would the AED give a "check patient" message?
A "check patient" message indicates that physical contact with the patient has occurred during the analysis phase or one of the AED electrodes has detached from the patient's chest. You must quickly remedy the problem so that the AED can analyze the patient's cardiac rhythm.

Question 4: What must you do after receiving a "no shock advised" message?
If the AED states "no shock advised," you should immediately resume CPR for 2 minutes and then reassess the patient. If the patient has a carotid pulse, you should assess breathing and continue to treat accordingly. If the patient does not have a carotid pulse, reanalyze the cardiac rhythm again.

Question 5: What should you do if this patient rearrests in your presence?
If the patient rearrests in your presence (witnessed cardiac arrest), you should immediately analyze his cardiac rhythm with the AED and deliver another shock if the AED advises you to do so. Following this shock, you should immediately perform CPR for 2 minutes, followed by assessment of the patient's pulse and reanalysis of his cardiac rhythm. Never remove the AED from a patient who has been resuscitated from cardiac arrest; they are still at a high risk for recurrent cardiac arrest.

Beyond eACLS Basics: How should you place the AED electrodes in patients with an automated implanted cardioverter/defibrillator (AICD)?
If the patient has an AICD or implanted pacemaker device, it will be palpable as a hard lump underneath the skin, typically on the patient's upper left chest. Placing the AED electrode directly over the implanted device may reduce the effectiveness of defibrillation. According to the American Heart Association, you should place the AED electrode at least 1 inch to the side of the implanted device.

eACLS Practice Case 5

A 65-year-old woman with a history of hypertension experiences a sudden onset of left-sided weakness, confusion, and slurred speech. Her daughter tells you that this began approximately 30 minutes ago. The pulse oximeter reads 98% on room air, therefore the patient is placed on oxygen with a nasal cannula at 4 L/min.

Question 1: Why is it important to establish the onset of symptoms in this patient?

____

____

The patient's blood pressure is 148/90 mm Hg. The pulse rate is 70 bpm and irregular, and respirations are 16 breaths per minute and unlabored. Further assessment of the patient reveals marked weakness to the left side of her body and a left-sided facial droop.

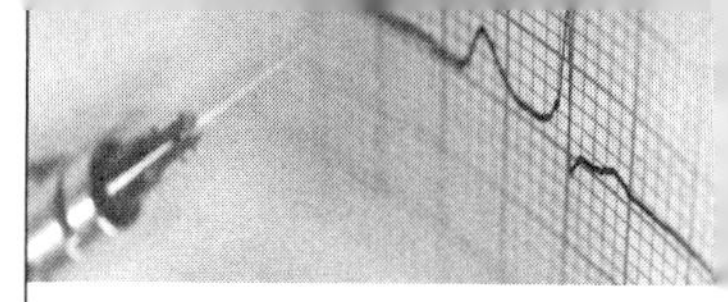

Question 2: What three physical signs may help you identify this patient's problem?

The patient is placed on a cardiac monitor, which reveals atrial fibrillation at a rate of 70 beats per minute. There are no signs of myocardial ischemia or injury on her 12-lead tracing.

Question 3: How could atrial fibrillation contribute to this patient's problem?

The patient remains conscious, although confused. An IV line of normal saline is established and set at a keep vein open rate. Blood is also drawn for chemistry and coagulation analysis.

Question 4: What blood test can quickly exclude a possible cause of this patient's problem?

The patient's condition remains unchanged. You notify receiving personnel of your impending arrival and apprise them of the patient's presentation, assessment findings, your interventions, and her present condition.

Question 5: What is the time frame for drug therapy after this patient reaches the hospital door?

The physician sees the patient within 10 minutes of arrival in the emergency department. Radiographic confirmation of her condition is obtained, and after the appropriate drug therapy is initiated, her neurologic deficits improve.

Beyond eACLS Basics: Why is D_5W contraindicated for this patient?

eACLS Practice Case 5 Summary

Question 1: Why is it important to establish the onset of symptoms in this patient?
This patient is displaying signs of an acute ischemic stroke. Establishing when the symptoms first began will determine (among other criteria) her eligibility for fibrinolytic therapy. Fibrinolytic therapy must be initiated within 3 hours after the onset of symptoms of a stroke.

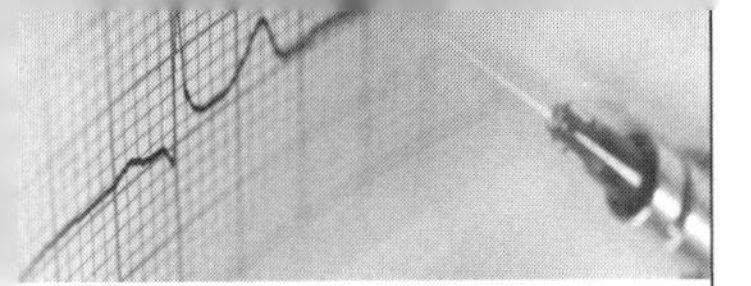

Question 2: What three physical signs may help you identify this patient's problem?
The Cincinnati Prehospital Stroke Scale identifies a potential stroke patient by assessing three physical findings: facial droop, motor arm drift, and speech difficulties. According to the American Heart Association, if a patient has an abnormality in any one of these three physical findings (as a new event), there is a 72% probability that they are suffering an acute ischemic stroke. If all three signs are abnormal, there is a greater than 85% probability of an acute ischemic stroke. Paramedics, nurses, and physicians can use the Cincinnati Prehospital Stroke Scale to determine the likelihood of a stroke.

Question 3: How could atrial fibrillation contribute to this patient's problem?
Atrial fibrillation can result in microemboli formation in the atria, which could travel to the brain and block a cerebral artery. Because of decreased atrial contractile force that accompanies atrial fibrillation, blood can stagnate in the atria, causing small clots.

Question 4: What blood test can quickly exclude a possible cause of this patient's problem?
Assessment of the patient's blood sugar level can exclude hypoglycemia, which can mimic certain signs of a stroke, such as confusion and slurred speech. You should routinely assess the blood sugar level of any patient with an altered mental status and administer dextrose if it is less than 70 mg/dL with signs and symptoms.

Question 5: What is the time frame for drug therapy after this patient reaches the hospital door?
The National Institute of Neurologic Disorders and Stroke recommended time target for fibrinolytic therapy initiation is within 60 minutes after the patient reaches the hospital door.

Beyond eACLS Basics: Why is D_5W contraindicated for this patient?
Hypotonic solutions such as D_5W are contraindicated in patients suspected of having a stroke because they can cause an abrupt fall in serum sodium levels and osmolality (concentration), as well as a shift of intravascular fluid that can result in cerebral edema and increased intracranial pressure.

eACLS Practice Case 6

A 48-year-old man presents with a feeling of "fluttering in his chest" that began 1 hour previous. He is conscious and alert and denies shortness of breath or chest pain. His blood pressure is 130/70 mm Hg. His pulse rate is 170 bpm and strong, and respirations are 16 breaths per minute and unlabored. The pulse oximeter reads 97% on room air.

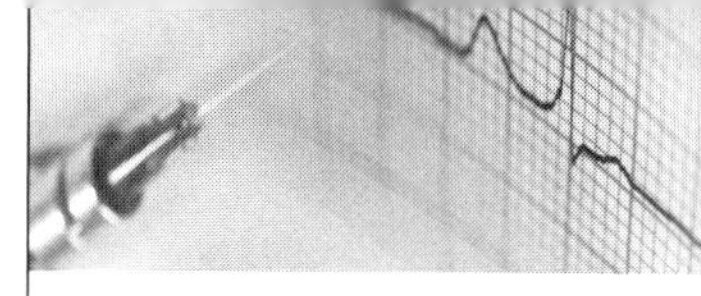

Question 1: What should your first intervention be for this patient?

The ECG leads are attached to the patient, and his cardiac rhythm is assessed (Figure 4-6). As your assistant is initiating an IV line of normal saline, you prepare to perform a therapeutic intervention.

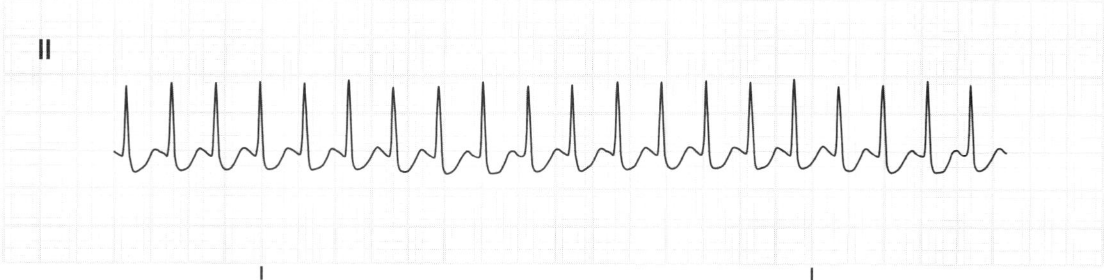

Figure 4-6: Your patient's cardiac rhythm.

Question 2: What intervention is used initially to slow this patient's heart rate?

After your initial intervention, the patient's condition and cardiac rhythm remain unchanged. Your assistant informs you that a patent IV line is now running. You open the medication box in preparation for your next intervention.

Question 3: What is the next treatment intervention for this patient?

The patient tells you that he has become short of breath. His skin is pale and diaphoretic, and his pulse is weak. You reassess his blood pressure and note that it is 84/50 mm Hg. After placing the patient on a higher concentration of oxygen, you prepare for further treatment. Your assistant hands you a syringe containing midazolam.

Question 4: What treatment intervention is indicated for this patient now?

After your next treatment intervention, you note a change in the patient's cardiac rhythm (Figure 4-7). His blood pressure is now 128/68 mm Hg. His heart rate is

76 bpm and is strong and regular, and his respirations are unlabored. He is no longer short of breath, and the pulse oximeter reads 98%.

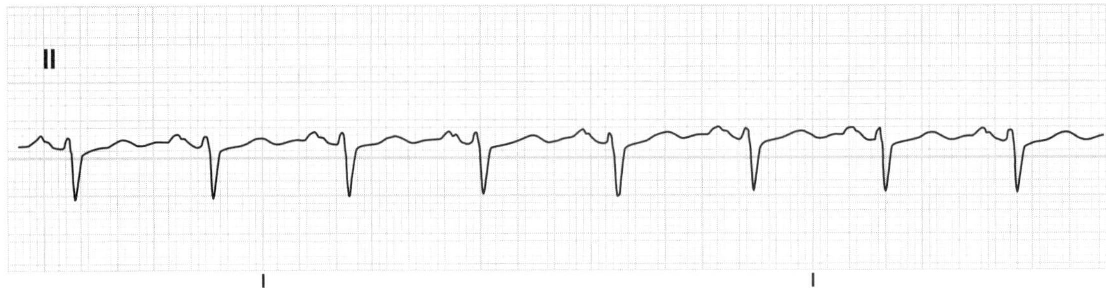

Figure 4-7: Your patient's cardiac rhythm has changed.

Question 5: How will you complete your treatment of this patient?

Once at the emergency department, a 12-lead ECG is obtained, which reveals a normal sinus rhythm, and blood is drawn to for electrolyte analysis. The patient's condition remains stable, and he is admitted to a telemetry unit for observation.

Beyond eACLS Basics: Why would multifocal atrial tachycardia NOT respond to synchronized cardioversion?

eACLS Practice Case 6 Summary

Question 1: What should your first intervention be for this patient?
Supplemental oxygen with a nasal cannula at 4 L/min would be appropriate for this patient. Because he is conscious and alert and not in respiratory distress and has an oxygen saturation of 97% on room air, he is not showing signs of hypoxia.

Question 2: What intervention is used initially to slow this patient's heart rate?
The patient is displaying a narrow complex tachycardia at 170–180 beats per minute. Because he is not exhibiting serious signs and symptoms linked to the tachycardia, he is stable. The initial intervention to slow the patient's heart rate is to perform vagal maneuvers. Techniques such as carotid sinus massage or the valsalva maneuver can be used.

Question 3: What is the next treatment intervention for this patient?
Because the patient remains stable and has not responded to vagal maneuvers, the next treatment of choice is to administer adenosine 6 mg via a rapid (over 1–3 seconds) IV push, followed by a 10 to 20 mL normal saline flush. Elevate the patient's arm to facilitate rapid delivery of the drug. If 6 mg of adenosine is unsuccessful, you may administer 12 mg, which can be repeated once, for a total dose of 30 mg of adenosine.

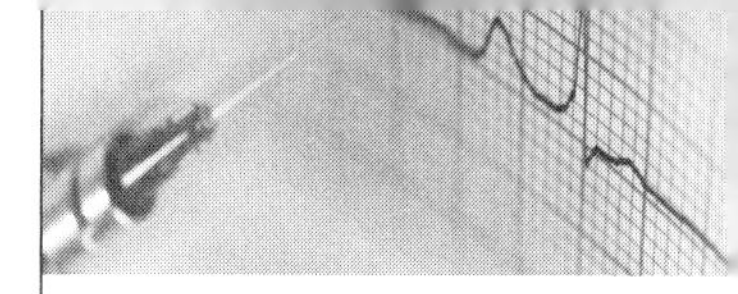

Question 4: What treatment intervention is indicated for this patient now?
This patient has developed serious signs and symptoms as the result of his narrow complex tachycardia and is therefore unstable. Treatment must now include synchronized cardioversion starting with 100 joules. Midazolam is used to sedate the patient before cardioversion. If 100 joules are unsuccessful in treating this patient, you should repeat cardioversion at 200, 300, and 360 joules.

Question 5: How will you complete your treatment of this patient?
You have successfully converted this patient's narrow complex tachycardia with cardioversion. He is presently in a normal sinus rhythm at a rate of approximately 80 beats per minute. It would now be appropriate to transport/transfer him for further care.

Beyond eACLS Basics: Why would multifocal atrial tachycardia NOT respond to synchronized cardioversion?

Multifocal atrial tachycardia and junctional tachycardia are both caused by an automatic or "irritable" atrial focus and will not respond to synchronized cardioversion. Rhythms such as paroxysmal supraventricular tachycardia are caused by a re-entry circuit within the AV junction and will generally respond well to cardioversion. Determining the underlying rhythm when a stable patient presents with a narrow complex tachycardia will enable you to select the appropriate treatment.

eACLS Practice Case 7

A 58-year-old woman complains of a sudden onset of substernal chest discomfort, nausea, and diaphoresis that began 2 hours ago. She tells you that she has coronary artery disease and has taken three nitroglycerin tablets without relief. Oxygen is placed at 4 L/min via a nasal cannula, and your assistant prepares to start an IV line of normal saline.

Question 1: Other than oxygen, what treatment can you provide to this patient without IV access?

____

____

The IV line is patent and running at a keep vein open rate. The patient's blood pressure is 148/90 mm Hg. Her pulse rate is 120 bpm and regular, and her respirations are 22 breaths per minute and unlabored. Your assistant attaches the ECG electrodes to the patient's chest and obtains a lead II cardiac strip (Figure 4-8). You prepare for your next intervention.

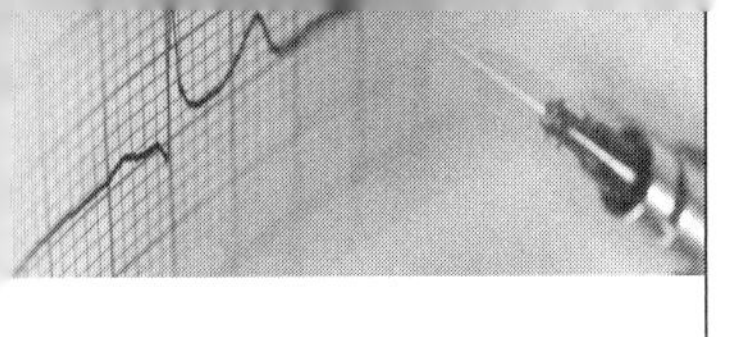

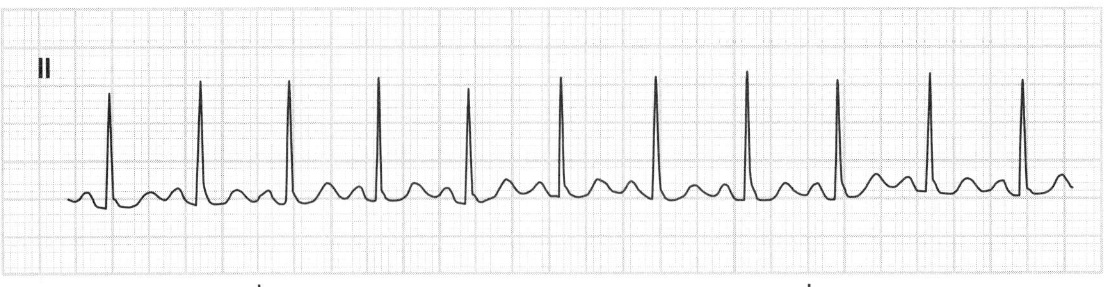

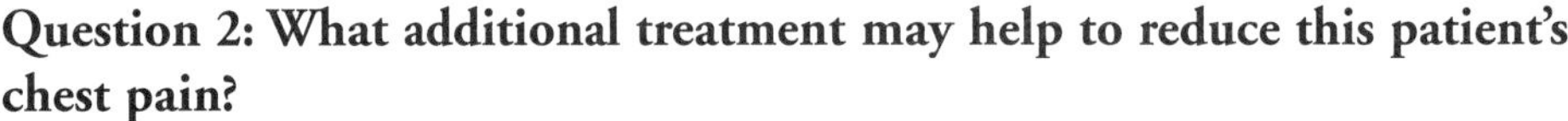

Figure 4-8: Your patient's cardiac rhythm.

Question 2: What additional treatment may help to reduce this patient's chest pain?

____

____

After your next treatment intervention, the patient tells you that her chest discomfort has improved somewhat. A 12-lead ECG tracing shows 3-mm ST segment elevation in leads II, III, and aVF. You ask the patient whether she has any known bleeding disorders or a stroke or recent surgeries.

Question 3: Why are you asking the patient these specific questions?

____

____

The patient denies a history of stroke, recent surgeries, or any bleeding disorders. She tells you that her chest discomfort is still present and is beginning to radiate to her jaw. You repeat her blood pressure, which is 130/70 mm Hg.

Question 4: Is further treatment required for this patient?

____

____

Reassessment of the patient reveals a blood pressure of 110/80 mm Hg, a pulse rate of 90 bpm and regular, and respirations of 18 breaths per minute and unlabored. She is still complaining of slight chest discomfort. You transfer/transport her to the emergency department for definitive care of her condition.

Question 5: What additional tests should you expect the emergency department physician to order?

____

____

After additional assessment and laboratory work, a definitive diagnosis of the patient's condition is quickly made in the emergency department, and within 30 min-

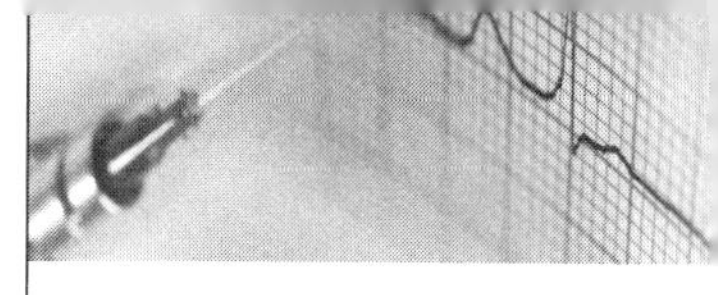

utes of her reaching the emergency department, the appropriate pharmacologic therapy is initiated. Within 20 minutes after this therapy is initiated, she is pain free.

Beyond eACLS Basics: How do fibrinolytic agents work to dissolve a thrombus?

eACLS Practice Case 7 Summary

Question 1: Other than oxygen, what treatment can you provide to this patient without IV access?
Aspirin (160–325 mg) should be given to patients with signs of an ACS as soon as possible. Aspirin has clearly demonstrated decreased mortality and morbidity from ACS and should not be withheld for the purpose of starting an IV line.

Question 2: What additional treatment may help reduce this patient's chest pain?
If three nitroglycerin tablets (or sprays) fail to relieve the patient's chest pain completely, you should administer 2–4 mg of morphine sulfate via a slow (over 1–5 minutes) IV push. You may repeat morphine in the same dose every 5–30 minutes as needed. Because morphine is a narcotic analgesic, you must monitor the patient for signs of central nervous system depression (e.g., decreased respirations, hypotension) and must be prepared to administer naloxone, a narcotic antagonist.

Question 3: Why are you asking the patient these specific questions?
These specific questions (among others) are asked to determine her eligibility for fibrinolytic therapy, which must be initiated with 12 hours after the onset of symptoms. She has already met the inclusion criteria for fibrinolytic therapy, which is ST segment elevation that is greater than or equal to 1 mm in two or more contiguous leads, signs of ACS, and the onset of symptoms within the last 12 hours.

Question 4: Is further treatment required for this patient?
Because the patient's blood pressure is stable and she is still complaining of chest discomfort, you should administer another dose of morphine (2–4 mg). Pain relief is an important aspect in the management of a patient with an ACS, as pain increases anxiety, thus increasing myocardial oxygen demand and consumption. This effect could extend (enlarge) her myocardial infarction and potentially cause cardiogenic shock or cardiac arrest.

Question 5: What additional tests should you expect the emergency department physician to order?
The impressive 12-lead findings clearly indicate inferior wall myocardial infarction; however, the physician will also obtain a chest x-ray, and blood samples to analyze her cardiac serum markers, blood chemistry, and coagulation times. Further questions will also be asked to confirm her candidacy for fibrinolytic therapy.

Beyond eACLS Basics: How do fibrinolytic agents work to dissolve a thrombus?
Fibrinolytic agents such as tissue plasminogen activator and streptokinase (Streptase) convert free plasminogen to the proteolytic enzyme plasmin. Plasmin in turn

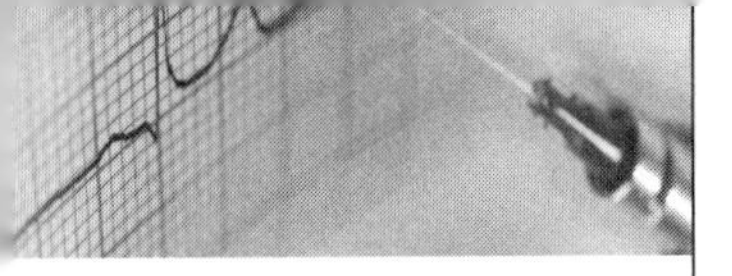

degrades the fibrin and fibrinogen matrix of the thrombus, thereby producing lysis (destruction) of the thrombus, hence the terms "thrombolysis" and "fibrinolysis."

eACLS Practice Case 8

A 49-year-old male suddenly collapses shortly after complaining of chest pain. The patient's wife says that he has had two previous heart attacks, and that he collapsed about 5 minutes prior to your arrival. Your assessment reveals that he is pulseless and apneic. Because his cardiac arrest was not witnessed, you perform 2 minutes of CPR and then assess his cardiac rhythm (Figure 4-9).

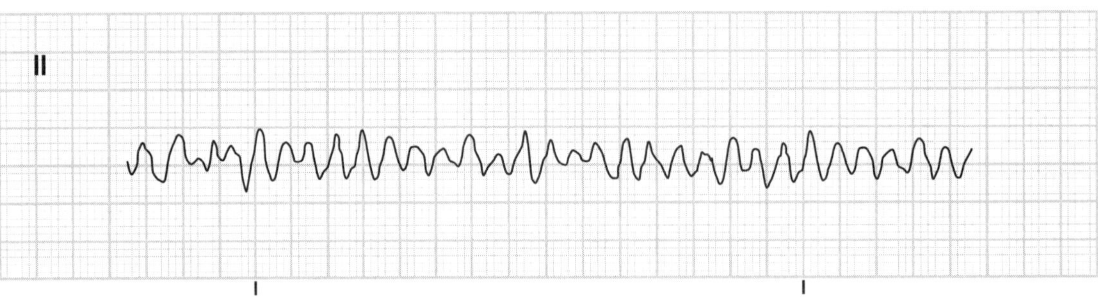

Figure 4-9: Your patient's cardiac rhythm.

Question 1: What immediate intervention is indicated for this patient?

____

____

Following your intervention, you immediately resume CPR. During this time, two assistants arrive to help you and your partner. An IV line of normal saline is established. Following 2 minutes of CPR, you reassess the patient and determine that his condition is unchanged. You repeat your previous intervention and immediately resume CPR.

Question 2: What pharmacologic intervention(s) should be given first?

____

____

The first medication is administered and circulated with effective CPR. Following 2 minutes of CPR, you reassess the patient and determine that his condition remains unchanged. The patient has also been successfully intubated.

Question 3: What intervention is indicated next for this patient?

____

____

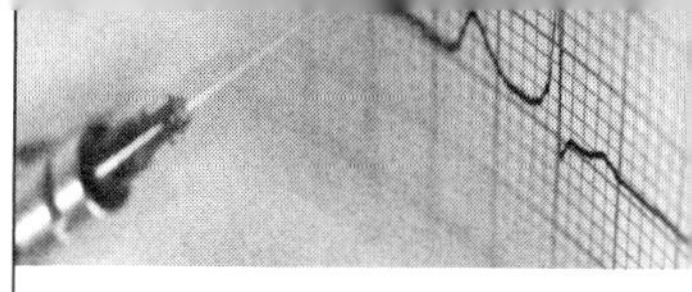

Following your next intervention, your two assistants immediately resume CPR. Your partner hands you the next medication indicated for this patient's condition.

Question 4: What pharmacologic intervention should be given next?

You administer the next pharmacologic agent for the patient while CPR is ongoing. After 2 minutes, you perform an electrical intervention and immediately resume CPR. After 2 minutes of CPR, you reassess the patient and note that his cardiac rhythm has changed (Figure 4-10). The patient now has a palpable carotid pulse.

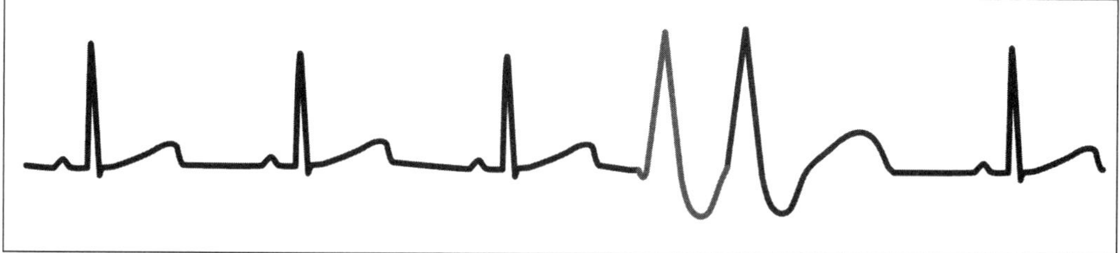

Figure 4-10: Your patient's cardiac rhythm has changed.

The patient remains apneic, so positive-pressure ventilations are continued. The patient's blood pressure is 100/70 mm Hg, and his heart rate is 76 beats per minute and irregular. You prepare an intervention to prevent a recurrence of his presenting dysrhythmia.

Question 5: What intervention will prevent a recurrence of this patient's presenting dysrhythmia?

The appropriate intervention has been performed. The patient's cardiac rhythm now shows a normal sinus rhythm at a rate of 70 beats per minute and no ectopy. His blood pressure remains stable, and the pulse oximetry reads 99% (intubated and receiving ventilations). You transport/transfer him for further stabilization of his condition.

Beyond eACLS Basics: What might this patient's presenting dysrhythmia have looked like if he had been hypomagnesemic?

eACLS Practice Case 8 Summary

Question 1: What immediate intervention is indicated for this patient?
This patient requires immediate defibrillation with 360 joules (or biphasic equivalent). He is in V-Fib, the most important treatment for which is prompt defibrillation. Ensure that no one is touching the patient before defibrillating. Following defibrillation, you should immediately resume CPR and reassess the patient's condition in 2 minutes.

Question 2: What pharmacologic intervention(s) should be given first?
One of two possible medications can be given to this patient as the initial pharmacologic intervention. Epinephrine 1 mg 1:10,000 via rapid IV push can be given. Vasopressin, in a one-time dose of 40 units, can be used to replace the first or second dose of epinephrine. Epinephrine is given every 3–5 minutes in a dose of 1 mg.

Question 3: What intervention is indicated next for this patient?
Because it has been 2 minutes since your last defibrillation attempt and the patient's condition has not changed, you must repeat defibrillation with 360 joules (or biphasic equivalent) and then immediately resume CPR for 2 minutes. After 2 minutes of CPR, reassess the patient and defibrillate again if needed.

Question 4: What pharmacologic intervention should be given next?
For refractory V-Fib or pulseless V-Tach, you can administer **one** of the following antiarrhythmic medications:

- Amiodarone: 300 mg via rapid IV push
  - Dilute amiodarone in 20–30 mL of D_5W before administration
  - Repeat in 3–5 minutes at 150 mg via rapid IV push
- Lidocaine: 1–1.5 mg/kg via rapid IV push
  - Repeat in 5–10 minutes at 0.5–0.75 mg/kg
  - Maximum dose is 3 mg/kg

Question 5: What intervention will prevent a recurrence of this patient's presenting dysrhythmia?
An antiarrhythmic maintenance infusion will help prevent a recurrence of V-Fib or pulseless V-Tach. Begin an infusion of the medication that aided in the conversion of the patient's ventricular dysrhythmia.

- Amiodarone (24-hour maintenance infusion)
  - 360 mg IV over the first 6 hours (1 mg/min) and then 540 mg IV over the remaining 18 hours (0.5 mg/min)
    - Maximum dose is 2.2 g per 24 hours

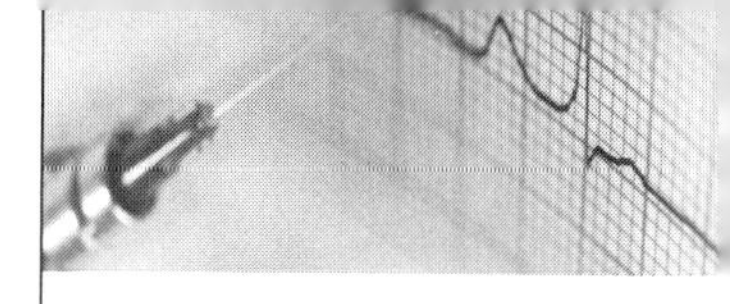

- Lidocaine
  - 1–4 mg/min titrated to the desired effect

Preventing recurrent V-Fib or pulseless V-Tach is a critical aspect of postresuscitation management. If the patient rearrests, the chances of a successful second resuscitation are lower.

Beyond eACLS Basics: What might this patient's presenting dysrhythmia have looked like if he had been hypomagnesemic?
Hypomagnesemia is a very common cause of polymorphic V-Tach, which in this patient, would have been treated with defibrillation, but magnesium sulfate 1–2 g IV would have been the preferred antiarrhythmic agent. Additionally, prolongation of the QT interval can cause Torsades de Pointes (TdP), a variant of polymorphic V-Tach. In these patients, you should avoid the use of medications that prolong the QT interval, such as procainamide.

eACLS Practice Case 9

CPR is in progress on a 70-year-old woman who was found unresponsive in her bed. There is no evidence of trauma. You instruct your team to temporarily cease CPR as you assess her cardiac rhythm (Figure 4-11).

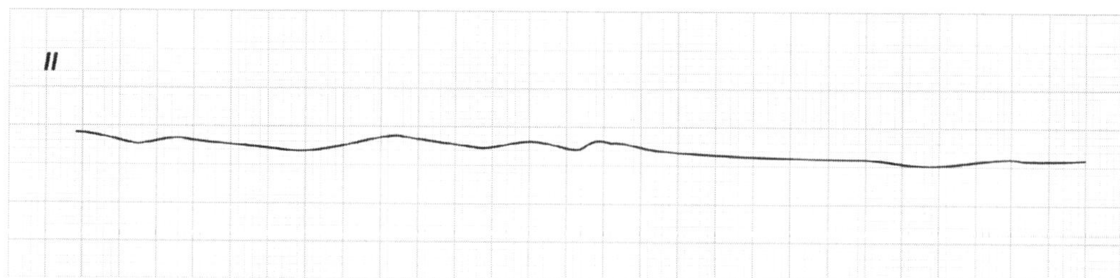

Figure 4-11: Your patient's cardiac rhythm.

Question 1: How will you confirm this patient's cardiac rhythm?

___

___

The patient's cardiac rhythm has been confirmed. CPR is continued and the ECG leads are attached. An IV line of normal saline has been established as attempts at ET intubation are being made.

Question 2: What pharmacologic agent(s) should be given to this patient first?

___

___

The first medication has been administered to the patient, whose condition and cardiac rhythm remain unchanged. As CPR is continued, one of your assistants tells you that the patient has been successfully intubated, and that ventilations are being performed at a rate of 8–10 breaths per minute.

Question 3: How would you treat acidosis as the cause of this patient's condition?

____

____

Measures are taken to treat the hypoxia and acidosis associated with the patient's condition. As other potential causes of her condition are excluded, you prepare for your next intervention.

Question 4: What treatment is indicated next for this patient's condition?

____

____

You have administered the maximum dose of the next intervention, and the patient's cardiac rhythm and condition remain unchanged. You have treated or excluded any possible causes of her problem. You elicit feedback from your team as to the cessation of resuscitative efforts.

Question 5: What factors should be considered when determining whether resuscitative efforts should cease?

____

____

You have exhausted all efforts at resuscitating this patient, and the decision is made to cease further resuscitative efforts. The patient's family is contacted and apprised of the situation. They agree with your decision.

Beyond eACLS Basics: Why is defibrillation not recommended for this patient's cardiac rhythm?

eACLS Practice Case 9 Summary

Question 1: How will you confirm this patient's cardiac rhythm?
When asystole presents on the cardiac monitor, you must assess another lead to ensure that it is not actually fine V-Fib. You should also increase the gain sensitivity on the cardiac monitor. If fine V-Fib is suspected or confirmed, defibrillate the patient at once.

Question 2: What pharmacologic agent(s) should be given to this patient first?
One of two possible medications can be given to this patient as the initial pharmacologic intervention. Epinephrine 1 mg 1:10,000 via rapid IV push can be given.

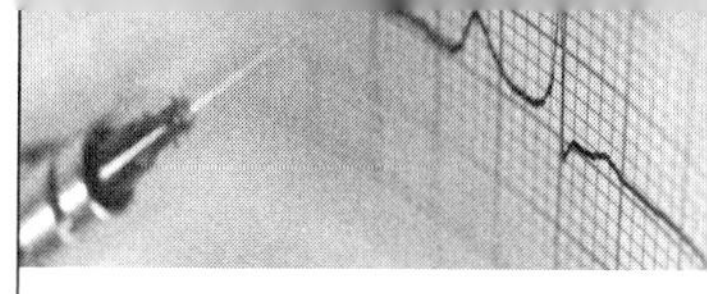

Vasopressin, in a one-time dose of 40 units, can be used to replace the first or second dose of epinephrine. If vasopressin is given as the first drug, you should wait approximately 10 minutes before initiating epinephrine therapy. Epinephrine is given every 3–5 minutes in a dose of 1 mg.

Question 3: How would you treat acidosis associated with this patient's condition?
Acidosis is present to some degree in all patients with cardiac arrest and worsens as the arrest remains uncorrected. Initial treatment for acidosis, regardless of the cause, is to ensure adequate oxygenation and ventilation. Measures should be taken, such as confirming correct tube placement and ensuring the delivery of 100% oxygen. Treatment with sodium bicarbonate 1 mEq/kg via an IV push should be considered 10 minutes after CPR has begun. If lactic acidosis is confirmed with an arterial blood gas, sodium bicarbonate should be given.

Question 4: What treatment is indicated next for this patient's condition?
The next intervention is to administer atropine 1 mg via rapid IV push. Atropine should be repeated every 3–5 minutes to a maximum vagolytic dose of 3 mg. Atropine is given to patients with asystole to exclude increased vagal tone as the cause of the asystole.

Question 5: What factors should be considered when determining whether resuscitative efforts should cease?
The American Heart Association recommends these criteria when determining whether to proceed with resuscitative efforts in a patient with asystole:

- Was acceptable BLS provided throughout the arrest?
- If V-Fib was present, was it eliminated?
- Was an advanced airway placed, confirmed, and maintained throughout the arrest?
- Was IV access established, with all rhythm-appropriate medications administered?
- Were potentially reversible causes of the asystole treated or excluded?
- Has asystole persisted for more than 10 minutes, after all appropriate therapies have been administered?
- Have family members been apprised of the situation?

Beyond eACLS Basics: Why is defibrillation not recommended for this patient's cardiac rhythm?
According to the American Heart Association, there are no valid data that suggest that routine defibrillation of asystolic patients yields a better outcome than without defibrillation. In fact, defibrillating asystolic patients can be harmful, as it can produce a "stunned" heart and profound parasympathetic discharge, thus eliminating

any possibility of restoring spontaneous cardiac electrical activity. Additionally, defibrillating asystolic patients can significantly reduce, if not eliminate, the chances of treating any potentially reversible underlying causes.

eACLS Practice Case 10

You arrive at the site about 5 minutes after a 55-year-old man collapsed. According to the patient's wife, he had been complaining of vomiting, diarrhea, and progressive weakness over the past 2 days. There is no history of trauma. Your initial assessment reveals that he is pale, pulseless, and apneic. After performing CPR for 2 minutes, you assess his cardiac rhythm (Figure 4-12).

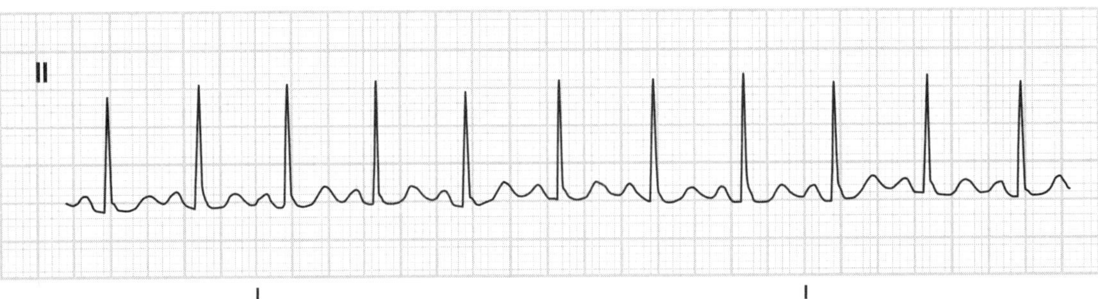

Figure 4-12: Your patient's cardiac rhythm.

Question 1: How would you define this patient's condition?

___

___

CPR is continued as a patent IV line of normal saline is established, and preparations for ET intubation are made. The patient's wife states that other than the recent illness, her husband is relatively healthy and takes no medications.

Question 2: What pharmacologic agent(s) should be given to this patient first?

___

___

The first medication for this patient's condition has been administered and is being circulated with effective CPR. The patient has been intubated, and your assistant reports clear and equal breath sounds and increased ventilatory compliance. Additional confirmation of proper tube placement is confirmed with capnography.

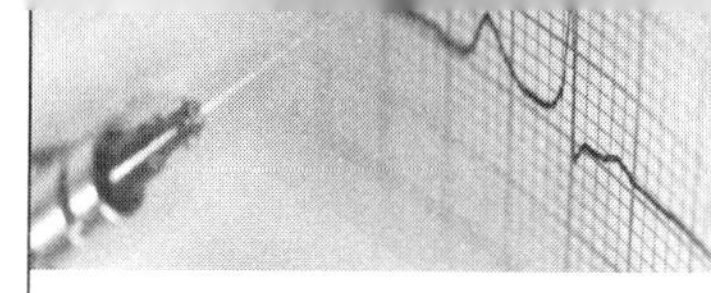

Question 3: Based on his presentation, what do you suspect to be the cause of this patient's condition?

A 500 mL bolus of normal saline is administered, and the patient is reassessed. He remains pulseless and apneic, with no change in his cardiac rhythm. Additional normal saline boluses are given as CPR is continued.

Question 4: Why would you NOT suspect a tension pneumothorax as the cause of this patient's condition?

After additional normal saline boluses, a carotid pulse is now palpable. You assess the patient's airway and continue ventilatory support. The patient's blood pressure is palpated at 70 mm Hg systolic. He is immediately transferred for further stabilization.

Question 5: What is commonly associated with the underlying cause of this patient's problem?

The patient continues to improve, and he is now in a normal sinus rhythm. After further stabilization in the emergency department, he is admitted to the medical intensive care unit and discharged home after a 10-day stay in the hospital.

Beyond eACLS Basics: What are the three "obstructive" causes of this patient's condition?

eACLS Practice Case 10 Summary

Question 1: How would you define this patient's condition?
This patient is in pulseless electrical activity (PEA). He has a cardiac rhythm (sinus tachycardia) on the monitor, but does not have a detectable pulse.

Question 2: What pharmacologic agent(s) should be given to this patient first?
One of two possible medications can be given to this patient as the initial pharmacologic intervention. Epinephrine 1 mg 1:10,000 via rapid IV push can be given. Vasopressin, in a one-time dose of 40 units, can be used to replace the first or second dose of epinephrine. Epinephrine is given every 3–5 minutes in a dose of 1 mg.

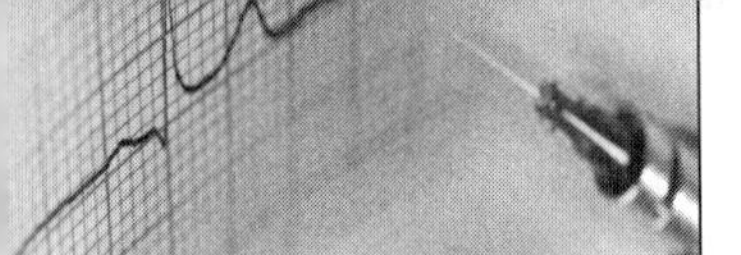

Question 3: Based on his presentation, what do you suspect to be the cause of this patient's condition?
With a 2-day history of severe vomiting and diarrhea, which has no doubt led to profound dehydration, you should be extremely suspicious for hypovolemia as the primary cause of his PEA. The narrow complex tachycardia and his pallor are also indicators of hypovolemic PEA. Hypovolemia is perhaps the most easily reversible cause of PEA, and thus, aggressive fluid resuscitation is needed with frequent reassessments of the patient. The American Heart Association states that it is acceptable to give an "empiric medical bolus" of 500 mL of normal saline, even without specific evidence of hypovolemia.

Question 4: Why would you NOT suspect a tension pneumothorax as the cause of this patient's condition?
The patient's breath sounds are clear and equal bilaterally, and your assistant is not having difficulty ventilating the patient (e.g., increased ventilatory compliance). A tension pneumothorax, although commonly associated with a narrow complex tachycardia, typically presents with a slow ventricular rate because of the accompanying hypoxia. This patient's history (e.g., no trauma) does not suggest the possibility of a tension pneumothorax.

Question 5: What is commonly associated with the underlying cause of this patient's problem?
Electrolyte depletion is frequently associated with severe dehydration. As water is lost from the body, so are electrolytes (e.g., sodium, potassium). Hypokalemia should be suspected when the T waves are flattened and prominent U waves exist. Although typically associated with wide QRS complexes, this patient is no doubt somewhat hypokalemic and hyponatremic, both of which need to be treated.

Beyond eACLS Basics: What are the three "obstructive" causes of this patient's condition?
The three obstructive causes of PEA are pneumothorax (tension), pericardial tamponade, and pulmonary embolism. The term "obstructive" means that blood flow is physically restricted (obstructed). A tension pneumothorax obstructs blood flow to the body because of myocardial and great vessel compression. A pericardial tamponade obstructs blood flow to the body as well because of myocardial compression caused by excessive blood or fluid in the pericardial sac. A pulmonary embolism obstructs blood flow to the lungs because of a blocked pulmonary artery.

Chapter 5

eACLS Practice Test

Introduction

This chapter contains a 50-question practice test that is designed to help you prepare for the final eACLS examination and to assist you in identifying potential weak areas. The questions in this practice test are similar to what you will encounter on the final eACLS examination. At the end of the practice test, you will find the correct answers and rationales.

To obtain a reliable assessment of your baseline knowledge of the material, it is recommended that you complete the practice test in its entirety and then refer to the correct answers and rationales.

____ 1. Immediate transcutaneous cardiac pacing (TCP) would be indicated for which of the following conditions?

a. Asymptomatic bradycardia.

b. Pulseless electrical activity.

c. Unstable ventricular tachycardia.

d. Complete heart block with hypotension.

____ 2. Which of the following statements regarding the AED is FALSE?

a. The AED will not analyze the patient's cardiac rhythm if movement is detected.

b. The AED will recognize ventricular fibrillation and pulseless ventricular tachycardia as shockable rhythms.

c. When the AED gives a "no shock advised" message, you have successfully restored a pulse.

d. The AED should be attached to the patient with unwitnessed cardiac arrest after 2 minutes of CPR.

____ 3. Which of the following medications would be indicated in the patient with a stable wide-complex tachycardia?

a. Atropine

b. Amiodarone

c. Morphine

d. Nitroglycerin

____ 4. A middle-aged woman presents with a narrow complex bradycardia. Her blood pressure is 80/40 mm Hg, and she is complaining of chest discomfort. You should first:

a. Start an IV and give atropine.

b. Obtain a 12-lead ECG tracing.

c. Give supplemental oxygen.

d. Begin a dopamine infusion.

____ 5. The Cincinnati Prehospital Stroke Scale consists of which of the following three assessment tests?

a. Facial droop, arm drift, abnormal speech

b. Arm drift, mental status, abnormal speech

c. Mental status, facial droop, blood pressure

d. Arm drift, facial droop, mental status

____ 6. Streptokinase falls under which of the following drug classifications?

a. Antiarrhythmic

b. Parasympatholytic

c. Fibrinolytic

d. Narcotic

Your patient presents with the following cardiac rhythm:

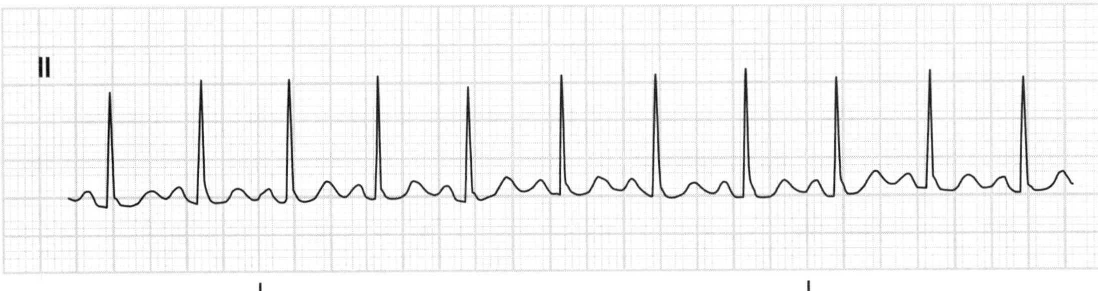

____ 7. Treatment for this cardiac rhythm should focus primarily on:

a. Synchronized cardioversion

b. Treatment of the cause of the rhythm

c. Administration of a normal saline bolus

d. Administration of a sedative drug

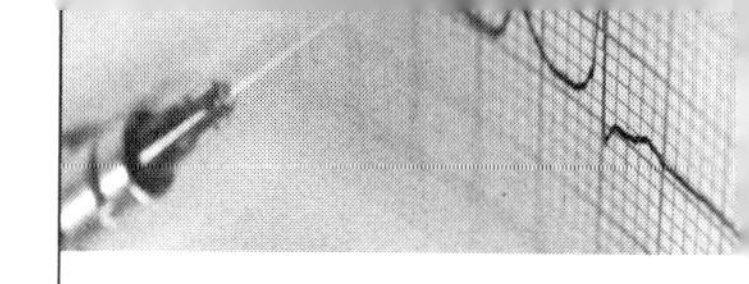

____ **8.** A 50-year-old male with a history of coronary artery disease presents with acute chest discomfort and nausea. After administering supplemental oxygen, you should next:

a. Give the patient 160–325 mg of aspirin.

b. Obtain a 12-lead ECG tracing.

c. Obtain intravenous access.

d. Give the patient nitroglycerin.

____ **9.** Which of the following medications will prolong the Q-T interval?

a. Epinephrine

b. Lidocaine

c. Magnesium

d. Procainamide

After performing 2 minutes of CPR on an older female patient whose cardiac arrest was unwitnessed, you note following cardiac dysrhythmia:

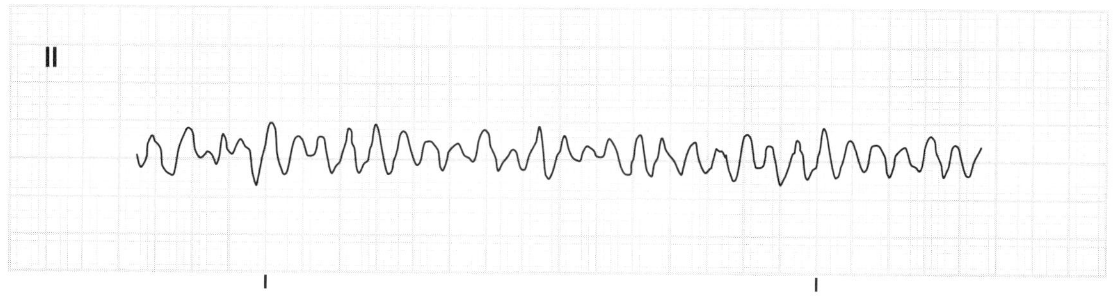

____ **10.** Your first action in treating the above cardiac rhythm is to:

a. Start an IV and administer epinephrine.

b. Defibrillate with 360 joules and continue CPR.

c. Perform immediate synchronized cardioversion.

d. Ensure that all contact with the patient has ceased.

____ **11.** Which of the following statements regarding vasopressin is TRUE?

a. Vasopressin is given to all adult cardiac arrest patients in a dose of 20 units every 3–5 minutes.

b. Vasopressin is used to replace the first or second dose of epinephrine for adult patients in cardiac arrest.

c. Vasopressin is the preferred initial drug to administer to adult patients with asystole or PEA.

d. Vasopressin should not be administered to adult patients with unwitnessed cardiac arrest.

_____ **12.** The recommended "door to drug" time for a patient with a suspected acute ischemic stroke is:

a. 10 minutes

b. 25 minutes

c. 45 minutes

d. 60 minutes

_____ **13.** You attempt ventilation of an unconscious, apneic patient but meet resistance and do not see the chest rise. Your initial corrective action for this problem is to:

a. Reposition the head.

b. Perform abdominal thrusts.

c. Perform chest compressions.

d. Perform endotracheal intubation.

_____ **14.** Patients in respiratory distress should be given oxygen in a concentration sufficient to maintain an oxygen saturation (SpO_2) of greater than:

a. 90%

b. 92%

c. 95%

d. 98%

_____ **15.** Normal saline fluid boluses have failed to increase the blood pressure in a patient with cardiogenic hypotension. Your next intervention should be:

a. Atropine

b. Epinephrine

c. Dopamine

d. Procainamide

_____ **16.** When should you perform 2 minutes of CPR before assessing a pulseless and apneic patient's cardiac rhythm?

a. If the patient has a known history of heart disease.

b. If the patient's cardiac arrest was not witnessed by you.

c. If the patient has an implantable cardioverter/defibrillator.

d. If you suspect the cause of the cardiac arrest was a massive stroke.

____ **17.** The AED has analyzed a cardiac arrest patient's rhythm and has given a "no shock advised" message. You should:

a. Immediately resume CPR for 2 minutes and reassess the patient.

b. Reanalyze the cardiac rhythm to confirm a nonshockable rhythm.

c. Assess for the presence of a carotid pulse for no greater than 10 seconds.

d. Discontinue chest compressions but resume positive-pressure ventilations.

____ **18.** Which of the following questions is of least significance when determining whether resuscitative efforts of a patient with asystole should cease?

a. Was adequate BLS performed throughout the arrest?

b. Were rhythm-appropriate drugs administered to the patient?

c. Has the family selected and notified the funeral home?

d. Was an advanced airway obtained and maintained?

____ **19.** Which of the following conditions is NOT classified and treated as PEA?

a. Pulseless idioventricular rhythm

b. Pulseless ventricular tachycardia

c. Pulseless sinus tachycardia

d. Pulseless second-degree heart block

____ **20.** Your goal in assessing a patient with a narrow complex tachycardia at a rate of 170 per minute is to:

a. Identify the presence of serious signs and symptoms.

b. Determine what medications the patient is taking.

c. Obtain a complete patient medical history.

d. Determine whether the patient has any medication allergies.

____ **21.** Which of the following drugs is used specifically to increase the patient's heart rate?

a. Epinephrine

b. Atropine

c. Dopamine

d. Amiodarone

____ **22.** A 60-year-old man is unconscious with a respiratory a rate of 6 breaths per minute and shallow. The cardiac monitor reveals a second-degree heart block at a rate of 38 beats per minute. Immediate treatment for this patient includes:

a. Doing transcutaneous cardiac pacing

b. Starting an IV line and giving atropine

c. Attaching an automated external defibrillator

d. Giving ventilatory assistance with a bag-valve mask

____ **23.** You have just performed synchronized cardioversion with 100 joules on a patient with an unstable wide complex tachycardia. You reassess him and note that his condition is unchanged. You should next:

a. Administer 150 mg of amiodarone.

b. Attempt transcutaneous cardiac pacing.

c. Repeat the cardioversion with 200 joules.

d. Begin an infusion of an antiarrhythmic drug.

____ **24.** Which of the following is NOT considered to be a serious sign or symptom?

a. Headache

b. Chest discomfort

c. Dyspnea on exertion

d. Altered mental status

____ **25.** A cardiac rhythm in which the appearance of the QRS complexes differ in shape and amplitude is said to be:

a. Monomorphic

b. Polymorphic

c. Supraventricular

d. Idioventricular

____ **26.** Midazolam is a medication that is commonly used for what purpose?

a. As an antiarrhythmic

b. Decreasing rapid heart rates

c. Increasing slow heart rates

d. Sedation before cardioversion

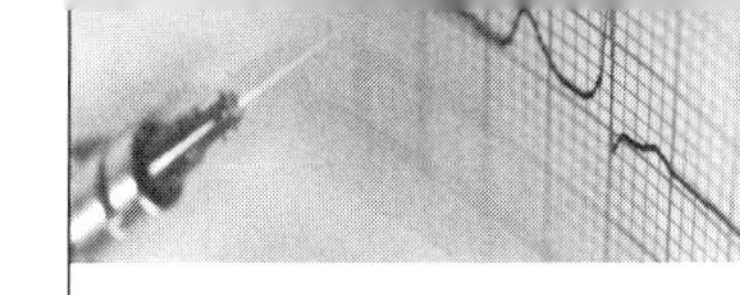

_____ **27.** Which of the following statements regarding narrow complex tachycardias is correct?

a. They typically originate in a location within the ventricles.

b. They are rarely associated with serious signs and symptoms.

c. They generally do not require cardioversion if the rate is less than 150.

d. They are always treated initially with adenosine, even if unstable.

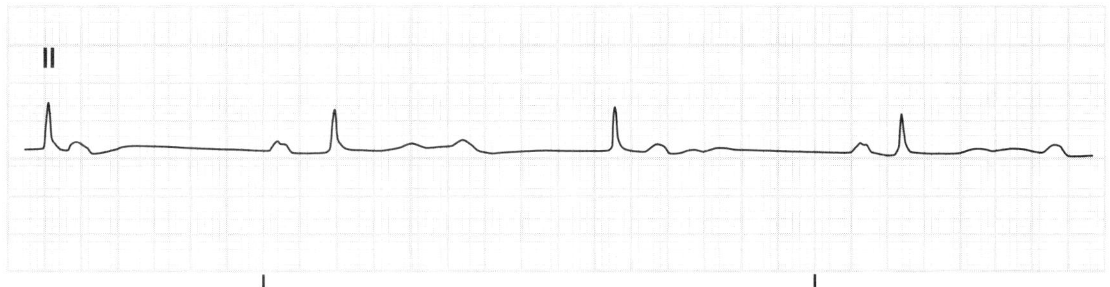

_____ **28.** You should interpret the above cardiac rhythm as

a. A third-degree AV block

b. Sinus bradycardia

c. A first-degree AV block

d. Idioventricular

_____ **29.** Which of the following is an example of a "relative" bradycardia?

a. A heart rate of 70 bpm and blood pressure of 110/70 mm Hg

b. A heart rate of 70 bpm and blood pressure of 80/40 mm Hg

c. A heart rate of 40 bpm and blood pressure of 70/50 mm Hg

d. A heart rate of 50 bpm and blood pressure of 120/70 mm Hg

_____ **30.** You have just defibrillated a patient in V-Fib. You look at the cardiac monitor and see what appears to be ventricular tachycardia. You should next:

a. Repeat the defibrillation.

b. Start an IV and give amiodarone.

c. Perform immediate cardioversion.

d. Perform CPR and reassess in 2 minutes.

____ **31.** The maximum adult dose for lidocaine is:

a. 1 mg/kg

b. 2 mg/kg

c. 3 mg/kg

d. 4 mg/kg

____ **32.** Diltiazem would be indicated for which of the following patients?

a. A 60-year-old male with atrial fibrillation

b. A 49-year-old female with ventricular fibrillation

c. A 52-year-old male with sinus bradycardia

d. A 72-year-old female with a third-degree heart block

____ **33.** A 40-year-old male with a narrow-complex tachycardia at 170 beats per minute has a stable blood pressure. You should give oxygen, start an IV line, and administer:

a. Cardioversion

b. Adenosine

c. Lidocaine

d. Atropine

____ **34.** Which of the following medications is MOST appropriate to administer to a patient with Torsade de Pointes?

a. Procainamide

b. Amiodarone

c. Magnesium

d. Lidocaine

____ **35.** All patients with a cardiovascular or respiratory system emergency will require oxygen, IV therapy, and:

a. Nitroglycerin

b. Endotracheal intubation

c. Cardiac monitoring

d. Early defibrillation

____ **36.** The correct energy setting for defibrillation for an adult patient is:

a. 100 joules monophasic or biphasic equivalent

b. 200 joules monophasic or biphasic equivalent

c. 300 joules monophasic or biphasic equivalent

d. 360 joules monophasic or biphasic equivalent

____ **37.** After attaching an AED to a patient in cardiac arrest, you push the analyze button and receive a "check patient" message. In addition to assessing for a carotid pulse and the presence of breathing, you should routinely:

a. Look for a medication patch.

b. Look for an implanted defibrillator.

c. Assess for medical alert bracelets.

d. Assess for correct electrode placement.

____ **38.** An older male is found unconscious and unresponsive. You must first:

a. Open his airway.

b. Assess for breathing.

c. Assess his cardiac rhythm.

d. Provide ventilatory support.

____ **39.** A common advanced alternative airway intervention in patients who cannot be endotracheally intubated is the:

a. Oropharyngeal airway

b. Needle cricothyrotomy

c. LMA

d. Pocket face mask device

____ **40.** After performing defibrillation with the AED, you perform 2 minutes of CPR, reanalyze the patient's cardiac rhythm, and receive a "no shock advised" message. This indicates that the patient is not:

a. in cardiopulmonary arrest.

b. in ventricular fibrillation.

c. breathing adequately.

d. in asystole or PEA.

____ **41.** A 56-year-old male is pulseless and apneic and presents with the following cardiac rhythm:

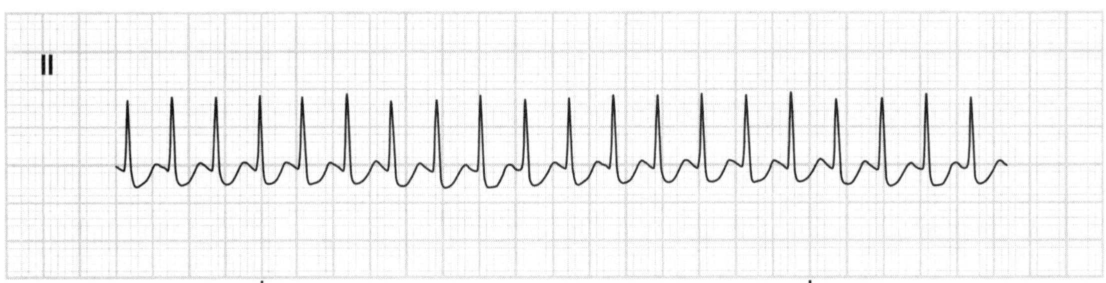

Treatment for this patient is likely to include which of the following:

a. Synchronized cardioversion

b. Adenosine 6-mg rapid IV push

c. Immediate defibrillation

d. Normal saline fluid boluses

____ **42.** A 60-year-old man complains of severe chest discomfort despite three nitroglycerin treatments. An IV line has been established, and his blood pressure is 148/90 mm Hg. Your most appropriate next treatment should be to:

a. Give 160–325 mg of aspirin.

b. Administer 2–4 mg of morphine.

c. Give the patient supplemental oxygen.

d. Begin an infusion of dopamine.

____ **43.** Ventricular fibrillation is a cardiac dysrhythmia that is most commonly seen:

a. Early in cardiac arrest

b. In patients with chest pain

c. In patients with a weak pulse

d. As a terminal event

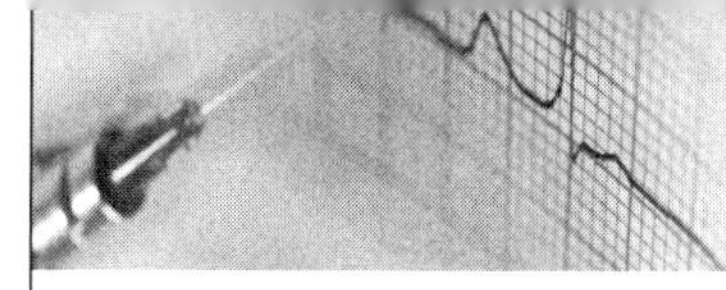

____ **44.** A 40-year-old female presents with a headache and the following rhythm:

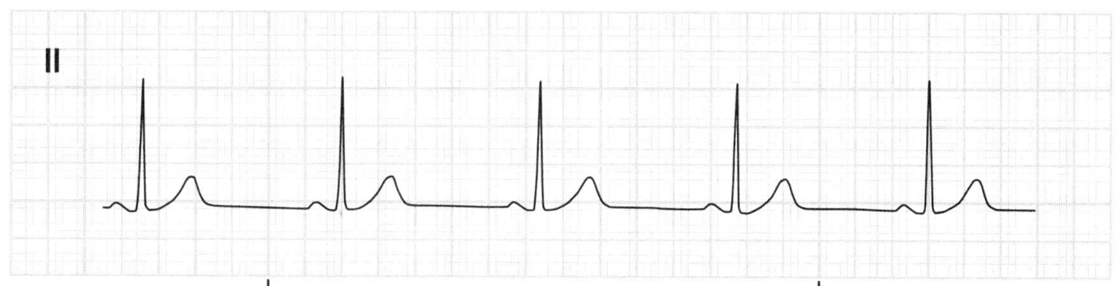

Her blood pressure is 118/58 mm Hg, and her pulse is strong. She is conscious and alert and denies chest pain or shortness of breath. Her treatment should consist of:

a. 0.5 mg of atropine

b. Transcutaneous cardiac pacing

c. Oxygen and careful monitoring

d. An infusion of epinephrine

____ **45.** Which of the following general statements regarding patient assessment is correct?

a. Treatment for a patient should be based on their blood pressure.

b. A careful and systematic assessment determines the need for treatment.

c. The absence of chest pain or discomfort means the patient is stable.

d. If a patient is conscious, they are breathing adequately.

____ **46.** Fibrinolytic therapy must be administered within how many hours after the onset of stroke symptoms?

a. 3

b. 5

c. 6

d. 12

____ **47.** Which of the following is NOT a common cause of conditions such as asystole and PEA?

a. Hypothermia

b. Hypovolemia

c. Hyperkalemia

d. Hyperglycemia

____ **48.** A 31-year-old male is in cardiac arrest. The cardiac rhythm shows a sinus bradycardia at 40 beats per minute. Assessment reveals absent breath sounds on the right side and jugular venous distention. Treatment for this patient's condition includes:

a. Delivering a 1,000-mL normal saline bolus

b. Giving higher than usual doses of epinephrine

c. Performing a needle chest decompression

d. Performing a needle pericardiocentesis

____ **49.** A 65-year-old female presents with cardiopulmonary arrest. She will require:

a. Defibrillation

b. Chest compressions

c. Atropine

d. Amiodarone

____ **50.** Which of the following medications would increase myocardial oxygen consumption and demand?

a. Oxygen

b. Atropine

c. Diltiazem

d. Adenosine

Answers and Rationales

1. **D.** TCP should be initiated as soon as possible for patient with symptomatic bradycardia, especially when accompanied by second degree type II or third-degree (complete) heart block. TCP is not indicated for patients with pulseless electrical activity. Unstable ventricular tachycardia is treated with synchronized cardioversion, not TCP.

2. **C.** When the AED gives a "no shock advised" message, this indicates that the AED has not detected a shockable rhythm. It does not indicate that the patient has a pulse. The AED will recognize two rhythms as being shockable: ventricular fibrillation and pulseless ventricular tachycardia. The AED will not analyze the patient's cardiac rhythm if it detects movement. If the patient's cardiac arrest was unwitnessed, especially if the arrest interval is greater than 5 minutes, you should perform 2 minutes of CPR before attaching the AED.

3. **B.** Medications used in the treatment of stable wide complex tachycardias include amiodarone, lidocaine, and procainamide. Atropine is used to treat symptomatic bradycardia. Both morphine and nitroglycerin are used to treat chest pain associated with acute coronary syndrome.

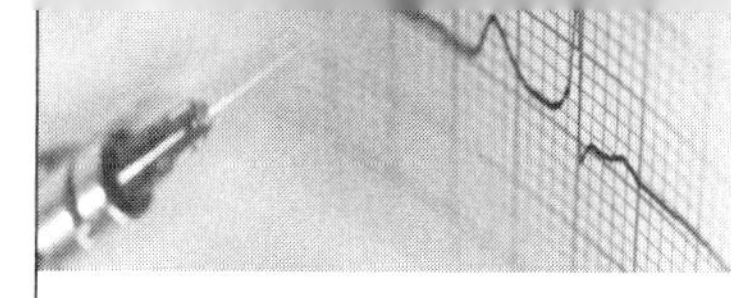

4. **C.** Oxygen is the first drug given to patients with a cardiovascular or respiratory system emergency. IV therapy, atropine, and a 12-lead ECG will all be necessary for this patient, but not before giving oxygen. A dopamine infusion may become necessary if other interventions are unsuccessful in treating her bradycardia and hypotension.

5. **A.** The Cincinnati Prehospital Stroke Scale consists of three assessment tests: facial droop, arm drift, and abnormal speech. Abnormality in any one of these three tests (as a new event) suggests a high probability of an acute ischemic stroke. Blood pressure and mental status assessment are not part of the Cincinnati Prehospital Stroke Scale.

6. **C.** Streptokinase (Streptase) is a fibrinolytic agent used to treat acute coronary syndromes, specifically acute myocardial infarction (AMI). Other fibrinolytics include reteplase (Retavase) and tissue plasminogen activator. Antiarrhythmic drugs include lidocaine and amiodarone. Atropine is an example of a parasympatholytic drug. Morphine is an example of a narcotic drug.

7. **B.** Sinus tachycardia is a manifestation of an underlying problem, such as fear, pain, hypoxia, or hypovolemia. A careful and systematic assessment must be performed in order to identify and treat the underlying cause, which may include normal saline boluses or the administration of a sedative drug. Narrow complex tachycardia with a ventricular rate of less than 150 beats per minute typically does not require synchronized cardioversion.

8. **A.** The American Heart Association recommends that patients with signs and symptoms of an acute coronary syndrome should be given 160–325 mg of aspirin as soon as possible. A 12-lead ECG, nitroglycerin, and IV therapy would all be appropriate for this patient as well, but not before giving aspirin.

9. **D.** Procainamide and amiodarone will both cause prolongation of the Q-T interval, which, on the cardiac monitor, represents the period of time between ventricular depolarization and repolarization. Epinephrine increases systemic vascular resistance and does not affect the Q-T interval. Lidocaine suppresses ventricular irritability with no effect on the Q-T interval. Magnesium is used to treat ventricular dysrhythmias associated with a prolonged Q-T interval (e.g., Torsades de Pointes).

10. **D.** This patient is in ventricular fibrillation and will clearly require defibrillation with 360 joules, followed immediately with CPR; however, you must ensure that no one is in contact with the patient first. An IV line and epinephrine are appropriate interventions for this patient, but not before defibrillation and CPR. Synchronized cardioversion is used to treat unstable wide or narrow complex tachycardias in patients who have a pulse.

11. **B.** Vasopressin can be used to replace the first or second dose of epinephrine for adult patients in cardiac arrest, regardless of the presenting cardiac rhythm. It is given in a *one-time dose* of 40 units via rapid IV push. There is insufficient evidence to support vasopressin as a superior drug to epinephrine and vice versa.

12. **D.** The National Institute of Neurologic Disorders and Stroke time targets for the patient with a possible acute ischemic stroke after reaching the hospital door are as follows:
    - Assessment by physician: 10 minutes
    - Availability of neurologic specialist: 15 minutes
    - CT scan (completed): 25 minutes
    - CT scan (formal reading): 45 minutes
    - Door to fibrinolytic therapy initiation: 60 minutes
    - Access to neurosurgical expertise: 2 hours
    - Admission to hospital bed (if receiving fibrinolytics): 3 hours

13. **A.** If your initial ventilatory attempt of an apneic patient is unsuccessful, you should first reposition the patient's head and reattempt to ventilate. If this is unsuccessful, you should perform chest compressions. Visualization of the airway (direct laryngoscopy) and removal of a foreign body airway obstruction with Magill forceps should be performed if chest compressions are unsuccessful. Endotracheal intubation may be necessary, but you must establish a patent airway first.

14. **A.** According to the American Heart Association, supplemental oxygen should be given in a concentration sufficient to maintain the patient's oxygen saturation (SpO_2) at greater than 90%.

15. **C.** Dopamine is indicated for hypotension, cardiogenic or otherwise, that is refractory to IV fluid boluses and is titrated to the desired effect. Atropine is used to treat symptomatic bradycardia. Epinephrine is an adjunct to atropine for symptomatic bradycardia. Procainamide is an antiarrhythmic drug that may exacerbate hypotension.

16. **B.** According to the American Heart Association, return of spontaneous circulation (ROSC) occurs more often in patients with unwitnessed cardiac arrest caused by ventricular fibrillation or pulseless ventricular tachycardia if 5 cycles (about 2 minutes) of CPR is performed before defibrillation. However, if the patient's cardiac arrest is witnessed by you, you should begin CPR and assess the patient's cardiac rhythm as soon as possible.

17. **A.** If the AED gives you a "no shock advised" message, you should immediately resume CPR and reassess the patient in 2 minutes. If, after 2 minutes of CPR, a pulse is felt, you should begin appropriate post-resuscitation care and

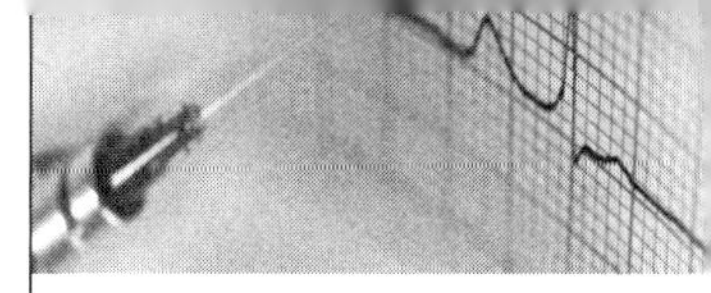

transport/transfer the patient immediately. AEDs have a high specificity for recognizing shockable rhythms; therefore, reanalyzing the patient's cardiac rhythm will only waste time.

18. **C.** Factors that should be considered when determining whether resuscitative efforts should cease include, among others, the performance of adequate BLS, the administration of rhythm-appropriate medications, obtaining and maintaining an advanced airway, and termination of V-Fib if present. You must ensure that the family is updated on the situation; however, it would not be appropriate to contact a funeral home until the patient is pronounced dead.

19. **B.** Pulseless ventricular tachycardia and ventricular fibrillation are both treated with immediate defibrillation and are not treated as PEA. All of the other choices listed are considered to be and are treated as PEA.

20. **A.** In order to provide the most appropriate treatment for the patient, your goal in assessing a patient with a potentially unstable cardiac rhythm is to determine the presence of serious signs and symptoms linked to his or her cardiac rhythm. Obtaining the patient's medical history, determining what medications the patient is taking, and ascertaining medication allergies are important aspects of assessing all patients.

21. **B.** Atropine is a parasympatholytic drug that is specifically used to increase the heart rate (positive chronotropy) of a patient with symptomatic bradycardia. Both dopamine and epinephrine possess chronotropic properties but are also used to increase myocardial contractility (positive inotropy). Amiodarone is used to control, among other conditions, rapid heart rates.

22. **D.** Control of airway and ventilation are your first priorities of care for any patient. This patient's bradycardia will clearly require atropine sulfate and/or transcutaneous cardiac pacing, but not before managing his airway. The AED is only attached to patients who are pulseless and apneic, which this patient is not.

23. **C.** If your initial attempt to cardiovert an unstable patient with either a wide or narrow complex tachycardia is unsuccessful, you should immediately repeat cardioversion with 200 joules. Antiarrhythmics (e.g., amiodarone, lidocaine, procainamide) would be appropriate if the patient were stable. An antiarrhythmic infusion is used to prevent a recurrent wide complex tachycardia after it has been successful with either an antiarrhythmic bolus or cardioversion.

24. **A.** Serious signs and symptoms include chest pain/discomfort, shortness of breath or dyspnea on exertion, jugular venous distention, altered mental status, and hypotension. Headache is not considered to be a serious sign or symptom.

25. B. A polymorphic rhythm (e.g. polymorphic V-Tach) has QRS complexes that differ in shape and amplitude (size). A monomorphic rhythm has QRS complexes that are all of the same shape and amplitude. A supraventricular rhythm indicates a cardiac rhythm that originates above (supra) the ventricles and typically has narrow QRS complexes. An idioventricular rhythm originates in the ventricles and is characterized by wide QRS complexes and a slow ventricular rate.

26. D. Midazolam (Versed) is a benzodiazepine drug that is used to induce sedation in patients before performing synchronized cardioversion. Examples of antiarrhythmic drugs include lidocaine and amiodarone. Drugs used to decrease rapid heart rates include adenosine and amiodarone. Drugs used to increase the heart rate include atropine and epinephrine.

27. C. Narrow complex tachycardias with rates of less than 150 bpm generally do not require immediate synchronized cardioversion because they are less commonly associated with serious signs and symptoms. A narrow complex tachycardia indicates a supraventricular origin, not ventricular. Narrow complex tachycardias (rates of more than 150 beats per minute) are commonly associated with serious signs and symptoms. Adenosine is used to treat a narrow complex tachycardia in stable patients.

28. A. A third-degree AV block is characterized by QRS complexes and P waves that are completely dissociated from each other and QRS complex widths of greater than 0.12 seconds. Sinus bradycardia has all components of a normal sinus rhythm; however, the ventricular rate is less than 60 bpm. First-degree AV block also has all of the components of a normal sinus rhythm; however, the PR interval is greater than 0.20 seconds. An idioventricular rhythm is characterized by wide, bizarre QRS complexes, absent P waves, and a slow ventricular rate.

29. B. Relative bradycardia is defined as a heart rate that is faster than one would expect relative to the patient's condition, usually their blood pressure. Absolute bradycardia is defined as a heart rate of less than 60 bpm. A heart rate of 70 bpm is somewhat faster than one would expect to see with a patient whose blood pressure is 80/40 mm Hg.

30. D. Immediately following defibrillation, you should perform CPR and reassess the patient's pulse and cardiac rhythm in 2 minutes. According to the American Heart Association, CPR should be immediately resumed for 2 minutes following defibrillation, even if a rhythm change is noted on the cardiac monitor. An additional 2-minute interval of CPR will help the heart recover from the arrest by improving cardiac output. Synchronized cardioversion is an appropriate treatment for unstable patients with a narrow or wide complex tachycardia who have a pulse.

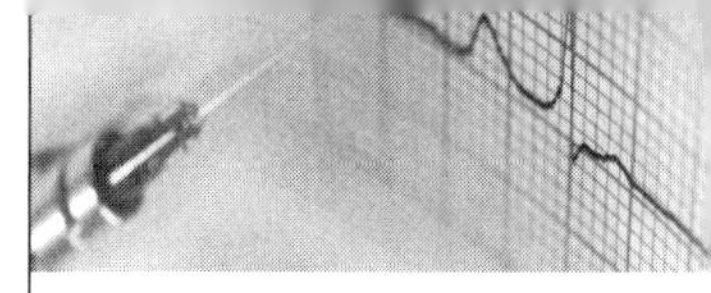

31. **C.** The maximum adult dose of lidocaine is 3 mg/kg.

32. **A.** Diltiazem (Cardizem) is a calcium channel-blocking drug that is used to control the rate of atrial fibrillation and atrial flutter and as an adjunct to adenosine for patients with stable narrow complex tachycardias. Patients with V-Fib need prompt defibrillation. Bradycardia, including sinus bradycardia and third-degree heart block, requires pacing and/or atropine.

33. **B.** Adenosine is given to hemodynamically stable patients with narrow complex tachycardias in an attempt to slow their heart rate and identify the underlying rhythm. Synchronized cardioversion would be appropriate if the patient's blood pressure was low or other serious signs and symptoms were present. Lidocaine is given to patients with wide complex tachycardias. Atropine is given to patients with bradycardia with serious signs and symptoms.

34. **C.** Torsades de Pointes (TdP), a variant of polymorphic ventricular tachycardia, is associated with a prolonged QT interval. Because hypomagnesemia is a common cause of QT interval prolongation and TdP, magnesium sulfate is the most appropriate medication to administer. Procainamide prolongs the QT interval and may exacerbate TdP, perhaps to the point of V-Fib; therefore, it is clearly not indicated. Amiodarone and lidocaine are indicated for polymorphic V-Tach with a normal QT interval.

35. **C.** All patients with a cardiovascular or respiratory system emergency will require oxygen, IV therapy, and cardiac monitoring. Cardiac dysrhythmias are common in patients with cardiovascular or respiratory system emergencies. Nitroglycerin would be indicated for patients with an acute coronary syndrome and adequate blood pressure. Patients who are in respiratory arrest would require endotracheal intubation. Early defibrillation is a critical therapy for patients with V-Fib and pulseless V-Tach.

36. **D.** The correct energy setting for monophasic defibrillation is 360 joules, both for the initial defibrillation and for all subsequent defibrillations. One defibrillation is performed after every 2 minutes of CPR for patients with V-Fib or pulseless V-Tach. Biphasic defibrillation uses lower energy settings, usually starting with 120–150 joules.

37. **D.** If the AED tells you to "check patient," it has detected that the patient is either moving (e.g., by a rescuer or spontaneously) or one or both of the AED electrodes is not properly placed. Looking for medication patches and implanted defibrillators would be appropriate actions before applying the AED. In general, all patients should be assessed for the presence of medical alert bracelets, not just those in cardiac arrest.

38. **A.** After determining that a patient is unconscious and unresponsive, your first action is to open the patient's airway and then assess for breathing. If the

patient is apneic or breathing inadequately, begin ventilatory support. Cardiac rhythm assessment is performed after airway and breathing problems have been addressed.

39. C. Common advanced alternatives to endotracheal intubation include the LMA and dual-lumen airway devices, such as the esophageal Combitube. The oropharyngeal airway is a basic airway adjunct that should be used during initial preintubation ventilations. The pocket face mask device is a common device for providing ventilations before performing endotracheal intubation.

40. B. A "no shock advised" message by the AED indicates that the patient is not in a shockable rhythm, such as V-Fib or pulseless V-Tach. It does not indicate that the patient is or is not in cardiac arrest. If you receive a "no shock advised" message, you should immediately resume CPR and reassess the patient in 2 minutes.

41. D. This patient is in PEA, a common cause of which is hypovolemia. Normal saline fluid boluses would be appropriate treatment for this patient. Narrow-complex fast cardiac rhythms that accompany PEA are often associated with hypovolemia. Adenosine would be appropriate if this patient had a pulse and was stable. Synchronized cardioversion would be appropriate if he had a pulse but was unstable. Defibrillation is performed on patients with V-Fib and pulseless V-Tach.

42. B. Morphine 2–4 mg via a slow IV push is appropriate if nitroglycerin fails to relieve completely the chest pain or discomfort associated with an ACS. Aspirin and oxygen therapy typically precede the use of nitroglycerin and morphine in patients with an ACS. Dopamine is indicated for severe, nonhypovolemic hypotension. This patient is not hypotensive.

43. A. Ventricular fibrillation is the most common dysrhythmia seen in early cardiac arrest and a pulse does not accompany it. In contrast to V-Fib, asystole is generally a terminal event with a high mortality rate.

44. C. This patient is not displaying serious signs and symptoms linked to her sinus bradycardia; therefore, she is considered to be stable. Her treatment should consist of supplemental oxygen and continuous careful monitoring. Interventions such as atropine, transcutaneous cardiac pacing, and an epinephrine infusion would be appropriate if she was unstable.

45. B. In order to provide the most appropriate treatment, you must perform a careful and systematic assessment of your patient, to include assessing airway and breathing, blood pressure, and the presence of serious signs and symptoms. Treatment decisions are not based on one sole parameter (e.g., blood pressure and chest pain). Just because a patient is conscious does not indicate that they are breathing adequately.

46. **A.** According to the American Heart Association, fibrinolytic therapy for a stroke patient must be administered within 3 hours after the onset of symptoms.

47. **D.** The "6 Hs" that represent the most common causes of asystole and PEA include hypovolemia, hypoxia, hydrogen ions (acidosis), hypokalemia, hyperkalemia, and hypoglycemia. Hyperglycemia is not a common cause of asystole or PEA.

48. **C.** This patient is in PEA because of a tension pneumothorax, and needs immediate chest decompression. Signs of a tension pneumothorax include unilaterally absent breath sounds, jugular venous distention, and as a later sign, tracheal deviation away from the affected side. A tension pneumothorax obstructs the flow of blood by compressing the myocardium and great vessels. This patient's problem is not hypovolemic in nature. Higher doses of epinephrine would be of no benefit to this patient. A needle pericardiocentesis is indicated for patients with a pericardial tamponade.

49. **B.** All patients in cardiac arrest will require chest compressions regardless of their presenting cardiac rhythm. The need for further treatment is based on their cardiac rhythm and may include defibrillation, atropine, or amiodarone.

50. **B.** Any medication that increases heart rate or myocardial contractility will increase myocardial oxygen consumption and demand. Such medications include atropine, epinephrine, and dopamine. Oxygen increases the myocardial oxygen supply. Drugs such as diltiazem and adenosine are used to decrease heart rate; therefore, they would cause a decrease in myocardial oxygen consumption and demand.

Notes

Notes

Notes

Notes

Notes

Notes

Notes